I Don't Go with **FAT** Boys

Weight Loss for People Who Love to Eat

Dr. Doug Pray
with Scott Smith

I Don't Go with Fat Boys: Weight Loss for People Who Love to Eat

ISBN: 0-88144-427-8

Copyright © 2009 by Dr. Doug Pray

Published by

Total Publishing and Media

9731 East 54th Street

Tulsa, OK 74146

www.TotalPublishingAndMedia.com

Doug Pray does a beautiful job of integrating his own struggle with weight loss with the development of a healthy means of dealing with this universal problem. His personal stories add credibility to his professional enthusiasm... His program is balanced and offers a scientifically and nutritionally healthy way to deal with the chronic problem of weight gain that affects so many people today. His faith, personal integrity, scientific knowledge and professional skills provide the context for an excellent book on healthy living that is both practical for everyone and professional in its expertise.

Dr. Robert D. Pierson, Executive Director, Leadership Nexus, Good Samaritan Church

This is a must read for anyone you love who struggles with their weight. Finally, a professional who truly understands the challenges of weight loss from both the patient and doctor's perspective. Doctor Pray's personal triumph over food addiction is absolutely inspiring! Its rare to find a book that makes you laugh out loud, choke with heartache, and then learn so much all in one read. This book is a true gift to anyone who has somebody in their life who struggles with these demons. Thank you for taking the time to write this book!

Dr. Jason M. Lord CEO Housecallrehab.com

"Obesity may soon be leading cause of preventable death in US. Unhealthy lifestyle choices become habits that eventually turn into unconscious behaviors and addictions in a cruel cycle. Most of the behaviors preceding the major causes of preventable death have begun by young adulthood. Dr. Pray has learned the secret to breaking the cycle of unhealthy choices. Based upon his personal experience, he charts a clear path that will lead you on your way to vibrant health, energy and longevity."

Mark Sanna, DC, ACRB Level II, FICC
President, Breakthrough Coaching

I Don't Go with **FAT** Boys

Weight Loss for People Who Love to Eat

For everyone who has ever been called a "fat boy," or girl.
…never again.

1

Humble Beginnings as a Fat Boy

The year was 1964. I was 11-years-old and in the sixth grade at Northeast Elementary School in Broken Arrow, Oklahoma. And I was madly in love with Paula Forbes.

I had always been crazy about girls, ever since I was a little kid. But Paula was different. She was special. She was so pretty and so mature for an 11-year-old. Back in those days, when a boy liked a girl as much as I liked Paula, he asked her to go steady. So one day while we were out on the playground at recess, I mustered up all my courage and asked Paula if she would go steady with me. She said yes! I gave her some kind of silly little ring (that probably came from a bubble gum machine), and Paula became my girlfriend. We were going steady.

I was on top of the world. I lived and breathed Paula. I dreamed about her during the day in school and at night in bed. The only time I ever saw her in person was in school or out on the playground. So when the school year drew to a close, I became depressed. Don't get me wrong – I loved summertime and my break from school, but that year, I didn't want summer to come because I knew I'd never see Paula.

But summer came anyway. In those days, boys didn't call girls on the telephone (at least not in Broken Arrow, Oklahoma). We didn't have cell phones, text messaging, or chat rooms, and the only tweets came from the birds outside. That summer, I literally never spoke to Paula. I thought about her every day.

That was the longest summer of my childhood. Three months crept by, and finally the new school year was just around the corner. I couldn't wait for school to start. I had never been so excited about the beginning of a new school year. I wanted to see Paula again more than anything.

On my first day of seventh grade at Oakcrest School, I didn't see Paula all morning. *What if her family moved away during the summer? What if I never see her again?* I was a nervous wreck. Finally, it was time for recess.

I ran out the playground, dodging the dodgeball game and leaping through a game of hopscotch. I had no time for games. I was on a mission. I had to find Paula.

Then I saw her on the other side of the playground. She was standing with two other girls, and although her back was to me, I recognized her immediately. I knew that was my Paula. My heart fluttered.

I ran up to Paula with a big, dumb grin on my face and tapped her on the shoulder.

"Paula, Paula, do you want to go steady again this year?" I asked.

She turned around, looked me up and down, and said, "Ew, I don't go with fat boys."

I was crushed. I had never experienced such harsh rejection. I didn't know what to say, so I didn't say anything. I just turned and walked away. For the rest of the day, I wallowed in my misery. I kept my head down on my desk during class. I took all I had to hold back the tears.

When I got home and saw my mom, the levee broke and my pent-up tears burst forth. I told my mom what Paula had said – that she didn't go with fat boys. Up until that moment, I didn't even realize that I was fat. I guess I had gained some weight over the summer, but I didn't notice. I was a kid. I didn't care if I had a little pudginess around the waistline. I simply never thought about it.

To make matters worse, my brother, who is 18 months older than I am, heard about what happened and gave me a nickname: *Fat Boy.* The nickname stuck for several years and really got under my skin. My brother was a skinny kid, and I was a Fat Boy, unworthy of a girlfriend. Pretty girls don't go with fat boys. I had learned this fact of life the hard way.

My mom, being an insightful mother, noticed how hard I was taking the unexpected break-up. Mom had a weight problem, too. She belonged to the TOPS club in Tulsa. TOPS stands for Taking Off Pounds Sensibly. It's a non-profit weight loss support organization that was founded in 1948.

The TOPS club is still in existence today. In fact, I recently spoke at their state convention. TOPS clubs across the nation educate members about nutrition and exercise. You can join a TOPS club in your area for low annual fee. The groups meet once a week to provide education, support, encouragement, and incentive to those who want to lose weight.

My mom took me to join the TOPS club in Broken Arrow. I guess she didn't want to take her son along to her own TOPS meetings. I didn't quite understand why then, but I understand now. Like other support group meetings, TOPS club meetings can get pretty personal. People talk about their weight problems as well as the issues behind them. My mom wanted us to have different support groups so that we could speak freely without fear of judging or being judged.

So, at age 12, I started going to TOPS meetings by myself. We met every Thursday night, and we had a weigh-in before the meeting. When the meeting started, if you lost weight, you called out, "I'm TOPS." If your weight stayed the same, you said, "I'm a turtle." And if you had gained weight during the past week, you had to announce, "I'm a pig." And, everyone said "Oink, oink!" They don't do that at meetings today, thank God times have changed. TOPS is a great organization. I'm thankful my mother introduced me.

The TOPS club taught me about accountability. You learn about accountability quickly when you have to say "I'm a pig" in front of a group of people! Such a practice may sound a bit cruel, but accountability is an important aspect of weight loss. When you have to answer to another person or a group about your eating habits, your exercise, and your weight loss efforts, you learn a lot more about yourself. The back-and-forth dialogue can reveal many epiphanies that you wouldn't experience otherwise.

TOPS also provided incentive to lose weight. My biggest incentive was the cash. Each week, everybody put some money in a pot. Whoever lost the most weight that week would win the cash pot. I won several times.

My mom provided added incentive. Whenever I lost weight, she would make the dinner of my choice. If I wanted to pig out on homemade brownies that night, that was okay – as long as I had lost weight that week. Looking back, that doesn't seem like the healthiest incentive program. But I guess it worked for me as a kid.

My mom and TOPS helped me lose a lot of weight. My first diet was the grapefruit diet. I simply ate a whole grapefruit before each meal. Many times, since I was in an inspired weight loss mode, I'd skip the meal after eating the grapefruit. I lost more weight than any kid in TOPS in the entire state. I lost 24 whole pounds. It may not sound like much, but that was a lot of weight for a 12-year-old!

Later that year, I was crowned the Tiny TOP Prince of Oklahoma. I received a crown, a robe, and an Oklahoma Tiny TOP Prince banner. I got an all-expense paid trip to the international TOPS convention in Toronto. When I walked down the aisle representing my state, hundreds of people cheered for me. It was a great feeling.

Suddenly I felt like a whole new person. I was no longer a Fat Boy. I was slim and confident. I went through several girlfriends. As for Paula – *Paula who?*

Little did I know, this was just the beginning a long stretch of yo-yo dieting and weight loss programs. My weight went up and down over and over again from then on out. I had gotten over Paula, but that fateful day on the playground affected my psyche at a deep level. After that day, I was always worried about being the Fat Boy. Even when I was skinny, I was worried about being fat.

When I started high school, I was extremely concerned about my weight. I was still crazy about girls, and I thought that every girl was thinking about how fat I was. Now, I look back at my high school photos and see that I was not overweight. It was all in my mind – but the mind is a powerful thing.

My confidence, which was sky-high when I was Tiny TOP Prince of Oklahoma, slowly faded as I got older. By the time I finished high school, my self-esteem was very low. I felt like I would be a paranoid Fat Boy for the rest of my life.

I married quickly – when I was 19. The marriage lasted for only a year, and I quickly married again. I was constantly concerned about my weight yet slowly gaining weight. I'd go on a diet, lose a few pounds, and then gain them all back plus a couple more.

Over the years, I tried over 100 diets. I got the same result with each one. I've lost at least 2,300 pounds in my lifetime. With each failed diet, I became a little more discouraged. *Maybe I'm just destined to be a Fat Boy for my entire life,* I'd think.

My second marriage lasted 17 years, and I blame my weight for my second divorce. My second wife was slim like a model – and beautiful like a model, too. When we divorced, she made a list of all the reasons why she wanted a divorce, including all of my faults. Guess what was on that list?

- *You're FAT!*

I felt the pain of Paula Forbes' playground proclamation all over again. This time around, I was truly heart-broken. I had lost my beautiful wife, my life partner of 17 years – not some girl on the playground who I only saw a few minutes a day during the school year. And my wife's ring didn't come from a bubble gum machine!

I lost a lot of weight after my second divorce. The irony is that I wasn't even very fat at the time. Sure, I was a little overweight, but at 6'1" and 230 pounds, I wasn't obese. But my wife thought I was fat, and she let me know. In my mind, I became Fat Boy all over again.

I stayed thin for a few years, but when the weight started to come back, as it always did, I lost all hope. I was the Fat Boy, and there was nothing I could do about it. What was the use in trying? I quickly ballooned up to 287 pounds. My waist got up to 48 inches. I was getting ready to buy my first 50-inch pair of pants when I decided, "I'm not going to do this!"

I should also mention that I was actually teaching nutrition at my local college when I gained all this weight. There I was standing in front of a classroom at nearly 300 pounds, lecturing about weight loss. Can you imagine how guilty I felt?

I had to do something. I was tired of feeling guilty, and I refused to buy 50-inch pants. I decided to try a new diet called the Atkins diet. I lost quite a bit of weight on this low-carb, high-protein diet. In fact, I was so impressed by the diet that I started teaching classes about it. I was a true Atkins aficionado.

Then a funny thing happened: My 17-year-old daughter introduced me to a whole new way of looking at nutrition. At the time, she was having some health problems, primarily due to hormone imbalances. She was also hypoglycemic. She'd have "weak attacks" when her blood sugar got too low. As the Atkins aficionado, I thought, "No problem! I'll fix her right up with my low-carb diet."

My daughter had other plans. She did her own research and discovered the book *Fasting and Eating for Health: A Medical Doctor's Program for Conquering Disease* by Joel Fuhrman, MD. After reading the book, my daughter informed me that she was going on a 21-day water fast, consuming absolutely nothing but water for three whole weeks.

"Are you crazy?" I asked her.

My daughter was undeterred, so I agreed to read Dr. Fuhrman's book. And, you know what, it all made sense to me. Sure, I was still skeptical, and some of Dr. Fuhrman's claims seemed a bit outlandish. For example, Dr. Fuhrman writes:

Therapeutic fasting accelerates the healing process and allows the body to recover from serious disease in a dramatically short period of time. In my practice I have seen fasting eliminate lupus and arthritis, remove chronic skin conditions such as psoriasis and eczema, heal the digestive tract in patients with ulcerative colitis and Crohn's disease, and quickly eliminate cardiovascular diseases such as high blood pressure and angina. In these cases the recoveries were permanent: fasting enabled longtime disease suffers to unchain themselves from their multiple toxic drugs and even eliminate the need for surgery, which was recommended to some of them as their only solution.

Despite my lingering doubts, I supported my daughter's decision. She was determined to go through with the fast, and I was determined to make sure she didn't damage her body in the process. We had blood work done before she started the fast, and I monitored her numbers throughout the entire three-week period.

During the fast, I checked on her constantly, which turned out to be an easy task. She basically lounged around and did nothing for three weeks. She didn't have the energy or strength to do anything. Near the end of the fast, she couldn't even read because her ability to focus had disappeared.

But she made it three weeks without consuming anything but water – and she lost a lot of weight. Additionally, the fast normalized her hormones and blood sugar level. She followed the advice in Dr. Fuhrman's book, and she healed herself. I was impressed – very impressed.

It wasn't long before my daughter bought a copy of Dr. Fuhrman's book *Eat to Live: The Revolutionary Formula for Fast and Sustained Weight Loss*.

"I'm going to start on this diet now, dad," she said, showing me the book.

She told me about the basics of Dr. Fuhrman's whole food diet.

"That won't work," I said smugly. "It's not a high-protein diet. In fact, it's almost all carbs. That won't work at all."

"Well, I'm going to do it, dad," she said. And I knew she would.

I was still teaching the Atkins diet, and my own daughter was going against my own advice. I was insulted! To make matters worse, since I wasn't exactly supporting my daughter, my new wife decided to go on the diet with her. Then I was even more insulted.

They went out and bought a bunch of nuts, seeds, fruits, vegetables, and beans. That night they made dinner and brought a plate into my office.

"Why are we eating this?" I protested. "It's all carbs! I can't believe you two are doing this!"

"Dad, just read the book," my daughter pleaded.

So I grabbed the book with the intention of picking it apart, critiquing it, and telling my wife and daughter everything that was wrong with it. With red ink pen in one hand and a fine-tooth comb in the other, I started reading.

I soon noticed that Dr. Fuhrman backed up all of his statements with research. I was so intent on proving him wrong that I looked up every single study he cited in *Eat to Live*. The harder I worked to prove him wrong, the more I agreed with his ideas. By the time I finished reading the book, I said, "You know what, this guy has it all figured out."

At that point, I had no choice: I had to try Dr. Fuhrman's whole food diet. I stopped counting carbs and started eating large salads. The results were amazing. I immediately dropped extra pounds and went down to near my ideal weight.

Then I made a big mistake: I went to a TOPS club meeting and told them that I would never be fat again. I told the members about Dr. Fuhrman's whole food diet. I told them that I had learned how to eat for the first time – that the whole food diet was God's diet plan for us all, the way we were designed to eat. Armed with this knowledge, I told them that I'd never be fat again.

Nine months later, I was fat again. The whole food diet worked for a while. Then Christmas came around. Since I was at my ideal weight, I decided that it was okay for me to have extra turkey and dressing. Then I reasoned that it was okay to have a piece of mom's homemade banana pie.

Mmm, that's good pie. One more piece can't hurt. After all, it's Christmas!

I gained a pound or two that week and a pound or two the next week. Over the next 90 days, I gained 30 pounds.

Looking in the mirror, I wondered how this could've happened. At the TOPS meeting, I said that I'd never be fat again. I had finally learned how to eat. Dr. Fuhrman's book gave me the perfect diet plan – and I still blew it. What happened?

That's when I realized that I was addicted to junk food – processed foods, refined foods, whatever you want to call them – high-calorie foods with low nutritional value. I started studying addiction and alcoholism, and I recognized the addictive patterns in my own life. I wasn't addicted to drugs or alcohol, but I certainly had a problem with high-fat, high-sugar food. I'm just as addicted to refined food as an alcoholic is addicted to booze.

I had to find a way to break the cycle of addiction. It's not just about knowing how to eat. If it were that simple, we'd all avoid junk food and not have any weight problems. The alcoholics who realize that alcohol is the source of their problems would simply quit drinking. But it's not that easy. We have to find some way to break the cycle of addiction.

At this point, I went back to Dr. Fuhrman's first book, *Fasting and Eating for Health*. I remembered how my daughter's fast had normalized her body's natural functions. It was almost as if the fast had rebooted her system. I wondered if a fast would help me to break my food addiction.

I learned everything that I could about fasting, cleansing, and detoxifying the body. I knew that I couldn't go on a three-week water fast. I had a business to run. I had patients to see and classes to teach. I had responsibilities that required my attention and energy. A shorter cleanse, however, would be feasible.

Working with a partner, Dr. Jeff Cartwright, I developed a healthy seven-day cleanse that allowed me to reap the benefits of a fast while maintaining my energy level. The program includes a cleansing formula to release toxins from nervous tissue and fat tissue; a metabolic boosting formula to enhance the body's ability to burn fat; and a meal replacement formula to maintain energy levels.

When I did my first cleanse a couple of years ago, I lost 13 pounds in seven days! My blood pressure dropped, my triglycerides dropped, my cholesterol dropped, and my blood sugar dropped. Best of all, I was able to break my addiction to junk food.

My cravings for burgers, fries, and cola disappeared. Before the cleanse, there was no way you could get me to eat a big bowl of fresh fruit or green vegetables because I was so addicted to junk food. That's all I craved and all I wanted to eat. After the cleanse, I didn't crave junk food anymore. I actually craved the steamed broccoli and other healthy foods.

Once I gave my body a chance to reboot itself, so to speak, my cravings changed; my body started to crave truly healthy food. My sense of taste changed, and the flavors of foods seemed to change. It was incredible! For the first time I could remember, eating healthy was actually easy and even enjoyable.

The modern American diet consists of refined foods that are full of toxins. Meats and dairy products contain pharmaceuticals, pesticides, and hormones. Processed foods contain all sorts of synthetic chemicals with names you can't pronounce. Even fresh fruits and vegetables are contaminated with toxins. And now we have to worry about genetically engineered foods that are introducing brand new inflammatory proteins into our bodies.

We're also exposed to toxins in the water we drink and the air we breathe. It's impossible to avoid toxins. The body does its best to process and eliminate toxins, but it can only handle so much. When you're taking in toxins faster than your body can process them, your body must store them in fat tissue. Your body fat is actually saving your life by holding onto to all those dangerous toxins!

Exposure to a high level of toxins – like the toxins in the typical American diet – overtaxes the body's natural defense system. The body is working so hard to process and store toxins that you don't have any energy left for important activities like exercise. However, when you detoxify and reduce your toxic load, your body can let go of the excess fat. There's no need for it any longer. After a cleanse, your fat will melt away, you'll have more energy, and you'll feel great.

After my first cleanse, I knew I was onto something big. I had broken my junk food addiction. But I also knew that, inevitably, the addiction would return as it always had. Addiction is cunning, baffling, and powerful. I had to develop a plan to keep the addiction at bay.

My plan revolves around accountability, mindfulness, careful monitoring of my weight, and quick action when the addiction begins to resurface.

Nobody's perfect. I'm certainly not perfect, and statistics show that I'm like most people. Over 98 percent of diets fail. Each year, Americans spend $60 billion on weight loss programs that have a two percent success rate.

Most people cannot follow a diet plan for long. A holiday rolls around, or they go out to eat, and they slip up. After gaining a few pounds, they become discouraged and eventually give up. I went through this cycle of yo-yo dieting for nearly 40 years before I realized how to make it work.

I monitor my weight carefully, and when I mess up

– when I gain a couple of pounds – I go on a mini-cleanse to nip the addiction in the bud. Instead of becoming discouraged, I lose the weight that I regained while keeping my body healthy.

I monitor my patients' weight carefully, too. My patients weigh-in each week. When patients gain a couple of pounds, I ask them what happened. If they went to a wedding over the weekend, perhaps they overate and gained an extra pound. I hold them accountable and encourage them to realize where they went wrong.

Then I tell them, "That's okay. I've done the same thing myself many times." Nobody's perfect. I offer them a solution: a mini-cleanse and a couple of days of strict adherence to the whole food diet. By the end of the week, they've lost the pound that they gained plus another. This system works, even for those of us who are not perfect.

Like many of you, I love to eat. It's my favorite thing to do. I love junk food, and I still eat it when I can. But I know how easily I become addicted to it again – and if that happens, then my cholesterol goes up, my triglycerides go up, my blood sugar goes up, my blood pressure goes up, I get fat, I get lazy, and I become discouraged. Suddenly, I'm addicted to junk food once again. I can't allow that to happen.

At the same time, I know that I will mess up, and that's okay. I try to stick to my whole food diet 90 percent of the time; 10 percent of the time, I allow myself to slip and eat junk food. I call it the 10 percent plan. Whenever I gain weight, a mini-cleanse resets my body chemistry before addiction can take hold. Then I go back to the whole food diet.

Instead of falling off the wagon, becoming discouraged, and reentering the cycle of addiction, my patients and I are able to continue moving forward without feeling guilty when we mess up. We never totally fall off the wagon.

Not everyone agrees with my weight loss plan. Some nutritionists feel that I'm allowing my patients to mess up. But guess what – people are going to mess up 98 percent of the time anyway. At least I have an answer and plan of action for them when they do. It's not a perfect weight loss plan, but it works for imperfect people like me.

This plan has provided the solution to my own weight loss problems, and it has worked for countless others as well. My patients have a 70 percent success rate for weight loss.

Most diets fail because people eventually get hungry and overeat or splurge on junk food. Here's the most important part of my weight loss plan: Never allow yourself to get hungry. Eat until you are stuffed. It's not how much you eat but what you eat that matters. That's where the whole food diet comes in.

Dr. Fuhrman has ranked foods according to their nutrient density. Nutrient density is the ratio of nutrients to calories. In ranking various foods, Dr. Fuhrman considers all the vitamins, nutrients, and phytonutrients (plant nutrients) in 1000 calories of the given food, then he assigns a nutrient density ranking of 1 to 1000. Here's a sample of Dr. Fuhrman's nutrient density scores from his website, drfuhrman.com: *(See Table on Next Page)*

Kale	1000	Tofu	86	Bananas	30
Collards	1000	Sweet Potatoes	83	Chicken Breast	27
Bok Choy	824	Apples	76	Eggs	27
Spinach	739	Peaches	73	Low Fat Yogurt, plain	26
Cabbage	481	Kidney Beans	71	Corn	25
Red Pepper	420	Green Peas	70	Almonds	25
Romaine Lettuce	389	Lentils	68	Whole Wheat Bread	25
Broccoli	342	Pineapple	64	Feta Cheese	21
Cauliflower	295	Avocado	64	Whole Milk	20
Green Peppers	258	Oatmeal	53	Ground Beef	20
Artichoke	244	Mangoes	51	White Pasta	18
Carrots	240	Cucumbers	50	White Bread	18
Asparagus	234	Soybeans	48	Peanut Butter	18
Strawberries	212	Sunflower Seeds	45	Apple Juice	16
Tomatoes	164	Brown Rice	41	Swiss Cheese	15
Plums	157	Salmon	39	Potato Chips	11
Blueberries	130	Shrimp	38	American Cheese	10
Iceberg Lettuce	110	Skim Milk	36	Vanilla Ice Cream	9
Orange	109	White Potatoes	31	French Fries	7
Cantaloupe	100	Grapes	31	Olive Oil	2
Flax Seeds	44	Walnuts	29	Cola	1

If you want to lose weight, you simply eat more nutrient-dense foods and avoid the foods with lower nutrient-density scores. It's that simple. Forget counting calories or carbs. Eat foods with a high ratio of nutrients to calories. You'll not only lose weight, but you'll also gain health.

Nutrient-dense whole foods contain proteins, fats, carbs, water, fiber, vitamins, minerals, and phytonutrients. Dark green, leafy vegetables like kale, collards, and spinach are the most nutrient-dense foods. Pop-eye had it right! You cannot eat too much spinach. In fact, the more spinach you eat, the more weight you'll lose. Each bite makes you healthier. You should try to eat a pound of raw leafy greens each day. You'll see amazing results.

A full pound of spinach contains only 100 calories.

You could eat 10 pounds of spinach every day and still lose weight (although I've never heard of anyone eating 10 pounds of spinach in a single day). That's the beauty of this plan: You never go hungry. You fill up on healthy foods and never allow yourself to get hungry.

Now, let's compare a pound of spinach to a pound of olive oil: One pound of olive oil has 2300 calories, and all of those calories come from 100% fat. Olive oil also contains some vitamins, but not in a quantity significant enough to raise its nutrient density score.

In recent years, olive oil has become popular among many dieters because of the Mediterranean diet. However, the Mediterranean diet works because of its focus on fruits, vegetables, and whole grains – not because of olive oil. Of course, olive oil, as a monosaturated fat, is healthier than saturated fats and polysaturated fats, but the fact remains that it's still extracted fat. If you're trying to lose weight, you should avoid excess oils and fats. We'll discuss the different types of fat in more detail in chapter 6.

When you study the nutrient density of foods, it soon becomes clear that God had a natural plan for us to remain healthy and thin naturally. The most nutrient-dense foods are also the lowest calorie foods. On the other hand, the most popular foods in the modern American diet are high in calories but low in nutrients. These foods are not natural. They have been refined, processed, and stripped of their nutritional value.

When you constantly eat foods devoid of nutritional value, your body craves more food to fill that void. That's why it's so easy to overeat and consume far too many calories when you're eating refined foods.

Most diets fail because the dieter's will power fails. Will power fails because people get hungry. My solution is simple: Don't let yourself get hungry! Eat, and eat until you're stuffed – but make sure that you're filling up on nutrient-dense foods.

My patients often call me in a panic after weeks of doing well in my weight loss program. "Help!" they say. "We're going out to eat at the steak house. What am I supposed to do?"

I tell them to plan ahead. Eat an apple before you go out to eat. The skin of an apple contains a natural appetite suppressant. It will help fill you up before you order at the restaurant, and you'll eat half as much.

When you order, start with a salad. Sometimes I even eat two salads when I go out to eat. I ask my server to leave off the croutons and add extra tomatoes, and I never choose a high-fat salad dressing. I usually order a low-fat balsamic dressing on the side. A healthy salad becomes unhealthy when you drown it in a high-fat dressing. Try to fill up on salad, and you won't want that slice of apple pie for dessert.

You can make healthy choices even when you're eating out in a restaurant. In a steak house, for instance, you can order the shrimp kabobs and a plain baked potato. After eating the apple, the salad, and the shrimp kabobs, you should feel satisfied. If you're still hungry, order another side of vegetables. Just don't allow yourself to get hungry.

Most popular diets work on the principle of calorie restriction, and dieters will eventually get hungry, overeat, and give up. A calorie restriction diet will help you lose weight if you stick to it, but how long will you stick to it?

Forget counting calories. Remember, what you're eating is more important than how much you're eating. Granted, you could lose weight on a pizza diet, a pasta diet, or even a chocolate diet if you restricted your calories.

If you're burning more calories than you consume, you'll lose weight. It's simple math. Here's the generic formula for weight loss based on calorie restriction: Multiply your current body weight times 10. If you weigh 200 pounds, the number would be 2,000; that's how many daily calories it takes to maintain your current weight. If you want to lose weight, cut your daily calorie intake by 400. By the end of the week, you will have lost a pound.

You can eat pizza three times a day, and if you're consuming 1,600 hundred calories or less with a current weight of 200 pounds, you'll still lose a pound a week. But the problem is that you'll eventually get hungry and eat more pizza. Your body will crave nutrients, and you'll overeat. With my plan, you don't have to count calories – and you don't have to go hungry.

In most cases, calorie-restriction diets actually promote weight gain. When people are on the diet, their metabolic rate slows down because they're eating less. When they go off the diet, their slower metabolism causes them to get even heavier than they were before they started the diet.

The Atkins diet revolves around counting carbs rather than calories. Carbs are severely restricted in the Atkins diet. Can you lose weight on the Atkins diet? Sure, but as soon as you go off the diet, you'll gain the weight back. In addition, the Atkins diet is not healthy. You're missing out on plant-based nutrients and health benefits.

The high-protein Atkins diet encourages consumption of meat products, and as you will learn from this book, a diet based on meat products has serious consequences for your health. Plant-based diets are much healthier. Plants not only provide the three energy producing macronutrients (protein, fat, and carbohydrates) as well as, vitamins, minerals, and water, but they also provide the essential micronutrients –phytonutrients.

Researchers are just now beginning to understand the importance of phytonutrients – natural chemicals that you can get only from consuming whole plant foods. Phytonutrients in fruits and vegetables act as powerful antioxidants; they neutralize free radicals in your body that cause oxidative damage and promote inflammation and aging. A plant-based diet will provide your body with everything you need to be healthy and prevent cancer, heart disease, diabetes, fibromyalgia, and other chronic diseases.

In searching for the perfect weight loss plan, I stumbled upon the perfect plan for holistic health. If you follow the advice in this book, you will not only lose weight but also reduce your risk of disease, extend your lifespan, and enjoy your new lease on life with more energy and vitality.

You will learn how to move right, eat right, and think right. If your head's not in the right place, then your weight loss is doomed from the beginning. A positive attitude is crucial. Successful weight loss is one-third diet, one-third exercise, and one-third mentality.

I understand your frustration. I feel your pain. I've been there myself. I will show you how to maintain a positive attitude even after you gain a couple of pounds. You don't have to fall back into the cycle of addiction. With a solid plan, you will overcome your addiction to junk food for good.

Like I said, not everyone agrees with my weight loss plan. Not everyone understands my weight loss plan. They don't understand what it's like to lose weight, gain it all back, go on another diet, lose weight, and gain it all back again. They're in that fortunate 2 percent of people who can stick to a healthy diet all the time. I'm in that 98 percent that will fail time after time, and that's why I developed this weight loss plan for imperfect people.

When I went on my first diet at age 12, I never imagined that I'd make a career out of weight loss. Now, weight loss is not just my career; it's my life's mission. Obesity is the biggest health threat in the United States. Approximately eight out of ten Americans are overweight, and nearly forty percent are approaching morbidly obese. That means your weight is literally killing you!

As a weight loss specialist, I feel as if I have to practice what I preach. I have overcome my addiction to refined foods, and I'm enjoying eating healthy, whole foods every day. My weight is down to 210 and slowly dropping even lower. With each bite of spinach, I become a little healthier.

I still love to eat, and I'll be the first to admit it: I still go out to eat and sample the junk food occasionally. But now I have a solid plan for when I mess up – and that plan is working so well for me that I want to share it with you.

It's time for a new beginning and a new life. Are you ready?

2

Our Toxic World (The Scary Chapter)

Have you ever watched House, M.D.? It's one of the most popular shows on television. Several episodes stress the importance of environmental health, which is overlooked all too often. Ironically, Dr. House frequently sends his interns to break into a patient's house. Now that's a dedicated physician.

But is breaking and entering really necessary? Is your home really that critical to your health? It certainly is - along with your work environment. (Note to my patients: Don't worry about me breaking into your home. I'm not as brave as Dr. House. But I will ask many questions about your environment and your lifestyle.)

Your environment and your lifestyle are the main determinants of your health. Of course, your genes play a role, too, but studies suggest that your environment plays a much larger role.

Most epidemiologists and cancer researchers agree that your environment accounts for 80 to 90 percent of your cancer risk, while genetics account for only 10 to 20 percent. In this context, environment includes diet, lifestyle, and exposure to toxins.

A toxin is a poison (usually a protein) produced by a living organism. Some animals produce toxins as predatory or defensive mechanisms. Snake venom, for example, contains a powerful neurotoxin capable of causing paralysis and death. Bacteria, fungi, and plants can also produce toxins.

When we humans produce toxic chemicals synthetically, they're technically known as a "toxicants." For the purposes of this discussion, we'll keep things simple and define a toxin as any poison that can cause disease.

Unfortunately, we live in a toxic world that's becoming more toxic every day. You may not even realize how toxic our world has become. To illustrate this point, I implore you to "play House" with me for a moment as we follow "John" through a typical morning in his life. Try to identify the toxins that might be responsible for John's headaches and chronic eczema that surfaced soon after he moved into his new apartment.

John wakes up when the alarm on his cell phone goes off at 7:00 a.m. Before he even opens his eyes, he scratches the rash on his neck. Yep, the eczema is still there. As he stretches, John gets a whiff the fresh paint on his walls.

John stumbles out of bed walks to the kitchen. He feels lucky to have gotten such a nice apartment. It was renovated just before he moved in. New carpet, new appliances, and a fresh coat of paint. John turns on the kitchen sink faucet, washes his hands with antibacterial soap, splashes his face, and takes a sip of water.

He opens the fridge and pours a bowl of fortified cereal and milk. He notices a small leak under the fridge and makes a mental note to call his landlord.

John tries to stay healthy and eat well. He slices a few strawberries to go with the cereal. Instead of sugar, he uses Equal to sweeten his coffee. He also has a small glass of cran-apple juice.

After breakfast, John heads to the bathroom for his

morning hygiene routine. He takes a hot shower using his new scented body wash. After drying off, he brushes his teeth, applies antiperspirant deodorant, and gets dressed. Since he expects to be working outdoors for part of the morning, John applies sunscreen to his face, neck, and forearms. You never can never be too careful, he thinks, especially when it comes to cancer.

John steps outside, takes a deep breath of smog, and immediately coughs. By the time he gets in his car to head to work, John's headache has returned, and his eczema is just as itchy as ever.

Did you notice any toxins that might be causing John's headaches and eczema? Some sources of toxins, like the smog, are fairly obvious. But some toxins are not so obvious. Let's examine some of the environmental toxins that might be causing John's symptoms.

John uses his cell phone as his alarm clock and keeps the phone near his body. Some studies suggest that electromagnetic radiation, particularly microwave radiation is toxic and increases the risk of cancer. Could John's headache be a symptom of a brain tumor?

Another study suggests that the microwave radiation from cell phones may increase one's sensitivity to certain allergens. Eczema is an allergic skin condition. Could John's cell phone be contributing to his eczema?

Could John's cell phone usage actually be causing his eczema? Perhaps. In 2008, the British Association of Dermatologists warned that "mobile phone dermatitis" was causing rashes on the cheeks and ears of many cell phone users. Most cases are caused by an allergic reaction to nickel-containing components.

While his cell phone could have caused John's eczema, dust mite allergen is the more likely culprit. Dust mites are microscopic arachnids that typically live inside bedding, as they love to munch on flakes of dead human skin. Note that

John scratched his neck as soon as he woke up. A typical mattress may house up to 10 million dust mites! Hot water kills dust mites - sunlight will do the trick, too - but it's difficult to wash a mattress or carry it outside for a sun bath. If you have allergies, impermeable dust mite covers will reduce dust mite populations in your mattresses.

The fresh paint and new carpet in John's renovated apartment area is likely releasing toxins into the air in the form of volatile organic compounds (VOCs). Paint, carpet, cleaning supplies, glues, plastics and building materials commonly emit VOCs. Many VOCs, like formaldehyde, are known carcinogens that can cause headaches, nosebleeds, and respiratory problems. Many home improvement stores now offer low-VOC or no-VOC paints so you can avoid these health ramifications.

John puts his health at risk even when he washes his hands. The antibacterial soap contains a chemical called triclosan, which has been shown to disrupt the endocrine function in laboratory animals. Researchers hypothesize that triclosan mimics thyroid hormone and binds to hormone receptor sites, blocking the genuine hormone from doing its job.

Furthermore, when triclosan combines with chlorine (which is added to nearly all municipal water supplies to kill germs), it forms chloroform gas, a probable human carcinogen. Oh yeah, John's toothpaste also contains triclosan. Does your toothpaste contain triclosan? Check the list of ingredients.

When John took a sip of water from the kitchen faucet, he swallowed some carcinogenic trihalomethanes (THMs). THMs represent yet another dangerous byproduct of the chlorination of water; they're formed when chlorine reacts with organic molecules in the water.

Biochemist Dr. Herbert Schwartz said, ""Chlorine is so dangerous that is should be banned. Putting chlorine in the water is like starting a time bomb. Cancer, heart trouble, premature senility, both mental and physical, are conditions attributable to chlorine-treated water supplies. It is making us grow old before our time by producing symptoms of aging such as hardening of the arteries. I believe if chlorine were now proposed for the first time to be used in drinking water it would be banned by the Food and Drug Administration."

So why are our public officials using such a dangerous chemical to kill the germs in our water supply, when safer and more effective alternatives are available? Well, that's the way it's always been done - and chlorine is cheap. By the way, John's morning sip of water also contained arsenic, lead, pesticide, phthalates, and a plethora of pharmaceuticals that had been flushed into the water supply, as well as a parasite called Cryptosporidium that's resistant to chlorine.

Now let's consider John's breakfast. At first glance, it appears to be rather healthy - fortified cereal, milk, strawberries, coffee with Equal, and apple juice. Unfortunately, this seemingly healthy breakfast consists of a chemical cocktail of toxins.

Any refined food that's "fortified" has been stripped of its original nutritional value to such an extent that extra nutrients had to be added. Dr. Fuhrman explains in Eat to Live:

Refining foods removes so much nutrition that our government requires that a few synthetic vitamins and minerals be added back. Such food is labeled as enriched or fortified. Whenever you see those words on a package, it means important nutrients are missing. Refining foods lowers the amount of hundreds of known nutrients, yet usually only five to ten are added back by fortification.

As we change food through processing and refining, we rob the food of certain health-supporting substances and often create unhealthy compounds, thus making it a more unfit food for human consumption. As a general rule of thumb: the closer we eat foods to their natural state, the healthier the food...

When you attempt to meet you micronutrient requirements with supplements or fortified products you miss those thousands of phytonutrients that accompany produce that is naturally nutrient rich. So every fortified food you eat is increasing your risk of cancer by decreasing your dietary intake of a food that could have supplied those calories in a more nutrient complete package. Fortified foods = processed foods. Processed foods = obesity and cancer epidemic.

The only truly fortified foods are whole foods. So what about John's strawberries? They're healthy, wholesome, and non-toxic, right? Well, it turns out that John purchased strawberries tainted with pesticides rather than organic strawberries. Strawberries appear on the Environmental Working Group's list of the "Dirty Dozen" most contaminated fruits and vegetables.

Here's the full Dirty Dozen list; when shopping for these 12 foods, it's best to buy the organic variety:

1. Peaches
2. Apples
3. Bell Peppers
4. Celery
5. Nectarines
6. Strawberries
7. Cherries
8. Kale
9. Lettuce
10. Grapes
11. Carrots
12. Pears

What about John's milk? Could it be toxic? Unless it's organic, it likely contains antibiotics as well as genetically engineered hormones. We'll discuss genetically modified foods in more detail later in this chapter.

While natural apple juice is non-toxic, most juice drinks

on the shelves are actually refined foods that are primarily water and high-fructose corn syrup (HFCS). John's cran-apple juice contains high fructose corn syrup, which likely plays a major role in the obesity epidemic. The "juice" also contains artificial colors and preservatives.

The Equal in John's coffee is made with the artificial sweetener aspartame (also in NutraSweet) , which accounts for over 75 percent of adverse reactions to food additives reported to the FDA. These reactions include seizure and death. Aspartame, a toxin that has been linked to leukemia and lymphoma, was actually classified as a "biochemical warfare agent" by the Pentagon at one point.

What about that small leak under John's refrigerator? Could that have anything to do with his headaches? Since John didn't move his refrigerator to check for standing water, he could have a large colony of mold growing under his fridge. Some molds produce toxins known as mycotoxins. Mycotoxins can cause headaches, as well as difficulty breathing, nosebleeds, memory loss, mood swings, and many other symptoms.

After breakfast, John took a shower. Water is clean and non-toxic, right? Wrong. John doesn't filter the chlorine out of his water. As the hot water formed steam, John inhaled chlorination byproducts like THMs. He also absorbed these chemicals through his skin. In fact, John's 15-minute shower exposed him to more toxins than drinking eight glasses of the same contaminated water.

John's scented body wash contains two other types of toxins - phthalates and parabens, both of which are suspected of disrupting the endocrine system. You won't see phthalates listed on the bottle; they're included under the vague term "fragrance." His antiperspirant deodorant contains parabens as well as aluminum. Even his stain-resistant shirt contains toxic formaldehyde.

What's next? Ah yes, the sunscreen. Most sunscreens contain toxic chemicals that are far more dangerous than the sun's rays. From free radical generators to estrogenic chemicals, many of these toxins are capable of crossing the skin barrier. Several studies suggest that sunscreen can actually increase the risk of cancer by blocking the production of beneficial vitamin D. Cancer researcher Dr. Gordon Ainsleigh believes that the pervasive use of sunscreen contributed to the 17% increase in breast cancer observed between 1981 and 1992.

There's nothing wrong with a healthy tan, in fact, it does a body good. But you should try to prevent your skin from burning; this is what could lead to skin cancer. I use sunscreen only when absolutely necessary. I try to prevent sunburn using common sense measures: hats, protective clothing, and not falling asleep by the pool.

When John walked outside, he got a lungful of smog and coughed. The microscopic particles in smog can damage the lungs as well as the heart.

Within 45 minutes of waking up, John has been exposed to dozens of toxins. Oh, I almost forgot, he also has toxic mercury in his dental fillings. Last year the FDA finally admitted that "silver" dental amalgams that contain mercury have neurotoxic effects.

So did you figure out what's causing John's headaches and eczema? With so many possible causes, it's impossible to know. The cause is likely a cumulative effect of all the toxins. Poor John. Poor us!

Do you remember Tim Burton's first Batman movie from 1989, starring Michael Keaton as Batman and Jack Nicholson as the Joker? In the film, the Joker appears on television to announce that he has poisoned Gotham City residents by placing chemicals in everyday products like deodorant, frozen dinners, shampoo, and cosmetics.

Batman realizes that it's not one single product but rather a mixture of certain products that's poisoning people: "There is a pattern - beauty products, personal hygiene… Somehow the Joker is supplying tainted ingredients at the source."

Once Batman figures out the pattern, the Joker resorts to other means of mayhem: "I feel it's time to expand the Joker line. I was askin' myself, what are the products that every consumer wants most? And that's when it hit me: the water you drink, and the air you breathe!"

Sometimes art mimics life a little too close for comfort. Twenty years after Batman hit theaters, I'm writing a book to warn you that you're being poisoned by a combination of toxins in the products you use, the water you drink, the air you breathe, and the food you eat.

You may not keel over immediately like the citizens of Gotham City, but if you're consuming a steady diet of toxins, you can rest assured that you're wreaking havoc in your body at the cellular level. It's not one particular toxin that's causing our health problems; rather, it's a combination of all the toxins that contribute to our body's total toxic load.

It kind of makes me wonder if the Joker is still out there somewhere, laughing.

The human body is well-equipped to process toxins. It has been dealing with natural toxins and invaders for thousands of years. But over 80,000 new chemicals have been introduced to our environment since World War II, and 1,000 more are added each year.

The liver, our body's main organ of detoxification, can only handle so much. Liver enzymes convert fat-soluble toxins to water-soluble molecules to be excreted in the urine and bile. The liver, however, is one very busy organ. It also aids in digestion, stores nutrients, and filters the blood to remove pathogens like viruses, bacteria, fungi, and parasites, among other functions. In our toxic world, the liver can easily become overwhelmed. When that happens, fat-soluble toxins must be stored in fat tissue - and that's when symptoms of disease begin to appear. Excess fat fans the flames of inflammation. Fat isn't simply an inactive blob of tissue; as you will learn in the next chapter, it pumps out hormones and inflammatory chemicals that set the stage for chronic diseases like heart disease and cancer.

Our Toxic Air

We can see the air pollution billowing out from smokestacks in big cities. Unfortunately, there's not a whole lot we can do about industrial air pollution as individuals. Cleaning up our environment will take years of political action. And you don't want me to get into politics here. Trust me.

But we can do something about the air in our homes and workplaces - and, according to the EPA, indoor air is typically two to five times more polluted than outdoor air. Sources of indoor air pollution include cigarette smoking, cooking, cleaning chemicals, nail polish, perfumes, glues, and paints. Pets bring dust, allergens, parasites, and bacteria into the home.

Ironically, the air-tight seals that make your home energy-efficient also make it an indoor air quality disaster zone. All of the pollutants get trapped indoors. Simply opening doors and windows periodically will improve your air quality. Obviously, you shouldn't smoke or allow others to smoke indoors. When you cook, turn on the ventilation fan. When you're working with paints, glues, or building materials that off-gas VOCs, do so outdoors, or wear a mask and open windows.

Vacuuming frequently will help keep your indoor air pollution at a minimum. You may also want to invest in a HEPA air purifier, especially if you have allergies or asthma. Certain plants remove toxic chemicals from the air, too. Aloe plants remove formaldehyde, peace lilies remove benzene, and spider plants filter out carbon monoxide.

Our Toxic Water

From added toxins like fluoride and chlorine to natural threats like parasites and heavy metals, water contamination poses serious health risks. The recent PBS Frontline documentary Poisoned Waters reveals that male fish in the Potomac River are producing eggs in their testes. Yes, that's right, male fish are producing eggs. Historically, egg production has been a job reserved for females.

Scientists have discovered similar "intersex" among amphibians as well. What's causing these bizarre intersex mutations? Sadly, the answer is human activity. We're flooding the environment with endocrine (hormone) disrupting chemicals. These toxins are everywhere - in personal care products, cleaning products, lawn care products, rubber products, plastic products, and other staples of human consumption. Most endocrine disruptors are petroleum-based chemicals that were developed during or since World War II.

Endocrine disruptors mimic natural hormones in the body. That's how they're causing the feminization of male fish in the Potomac. These chemicals not only disrupt estrogen and testosterone levels, but they also disrupt thyroid function, reproductive function, and immune system function.

In fact, nobody really knows how much damage these chemicals are causing – because, according to Poisoned Waters, even the EPA doesn't know how to measure, much less regulate, many of these new chemicals – but scientists do know that they are extremely powerful at infinitesimally small quantities. It doesn't take much poison to cause a male fish to start producing caviar.

"The long-term, slow-motion risk is already being spelled out in epidemiologic data, studies – large population studies," said Dr. Robert Lawrence of the Johns Hopkins School of Public Health in the documentary.

"There are 5 million people being exposed to endocrine disruptors just in the Mid-Atlantic region, and yet we don't know precisely how many of them are going to develop premature breast cancer, going to have problems with reproduction, going to have all kinds of congenital anomalies of the male genitalia, things that are happening at a broad low level so that they don't raise the alarm in the general public."

Again, the EPA does not regulate these chemicals because they don't even know how to measure many of them. Water treatment is not intended to remove these chemicals, and according to the film, tests show that about 2/3 of them are still in drinking water after the treatment process.

In other news, the EPA recently decided not to regulate perchlorate, a rocket fuel ingredient that interferes with thyroid function. According to the Environmental Working Group, perchlorate contaminates the water supply of at least 20 million Americans in at least 43 states. Yep, we're drinking rocket fuel. Great.

Just seven years ago, the EPA wanted to regulate perchlorate in the water. The agency suggested a limit for perchlorate contamination after they found that even small reductions in thyroid function in infants can lower IQ and cause behavioral problems.

Here's the rub: The source of all that rocket fuel in our drinking water is the Defense Department – from decades of testing missiles and rockets – and the Pentagon would face hundreds of millions of dollars in cleanup costs if perchlorate were regulated. And so the EPA called off its six-year effort to regulate the chemical in September 2008.

I recommend a home drinking water filter as well as a shower filter (unless you enjoy the taste of rocket fuel).

Our Toxic Products

Everything comes wrapped in plastic. You can't get away from it. All the plastic that has ever been made is still here, piling up in our landfills and oceans. And now it's inside of us. Most Americans are literally urinating plastic on a daily basis.

Last year a CDC analysis estimated that bisphenol-A (BPA) is now detectable in the blood of 93% of Americans.

BPA is a toxin found in a wide array of plastics, from canned food linings to the coating on children's teeth. BPA, like so many other synthetic chemicals, disrupts the endocrine system by mimicking estrogen. It has been linked to early puberty, heart disease, and diabetes.

Personal care products and cosmetic products act as vehicles for thousands of hidden toxins. Toxicologist Dr. Tim Kropp of the Environmental Working Group (EWG) explains, "Most of the products you use have chemicals that haven't been tested for safety at all . . . Most people assume that if you see something on the shelf, it's safe for you. The findings of our study really contradict that."

The 2004 EWG study examined 14,000 common personal care products and cosmetics. Over 46% of the products contained ingredients that may contribute to birth defects. Over 44% of these products contained chemicals that are possible human carcinogens, and nearly 86% of the products contained ingredients that may cause allergic reactions.

Toxins lurk on every shelf. I'm sure you remember the tainted dog food recall of 2007. Hundreds of dogs died after eating food contaminated with melamine, an industrial chemical that can cause kidney failure.

Not even children's toys are safe from contamination. The Ecology Center conducted a study in 2008 and found that toys are commonly contaminated with lead, mercury, arsenic, and other poisons.

"When you see these toys sitting on the shelf, there is no way to determine which products are made with toxic chemicals and which aren't," Mike Shriberg, policy director of the Ecology Center, told Forbes. "They cost the same amount and look the same. It really shows that manufacturers have no excuse for making toys with dangerous chemicals."

Children's jewelry is the worst offender. "Toxins were five times as likely to be found in jewelry as any other category of children's products," said Shriberg. In February 2006, a four-year-old boy in Minnesota died after accidentally swallowing a heart-shaped toy jewelry locket that contained toxic levels of lead.

And let's not forget the most toxic products of all: pharmaceuticals. Pharmaceuticals are, by nature, toxic chemicals. Let me make it clear that I'm not totally against the use of medicine; medicine saves lives. But I'm willing to bet that the pharmaceutical industry does more harm than good. Hospitals, for example, flush 250 million pounds of toxic drugs down the toilet each year. Those drugs end up in our water and food.

Many people don't realize that even common over-the-counter medicines can be extremely toxic and deadly. Acetaminophen (Tylenol), for example, can easily cause kidney damage, liver damage, and death when taken in excessive quantity. Tylenol overdose kills about 500 people each year. To be safe, never drink alcohol if you're taking medication, and always read medication warnings.

Our Toxic Food

Here's the single most important piece of advice in this whole book: If you want to lose weight and get healthy, stop eating fake food and start eating real food.

What do I mean by "fake" food? Refined food, processed food, treated food, fortified food, genetically modified food, food injected with artificial colors, fragrances, aromas, and preservatives - essentially 95 percent of the food that lines the shelves in grocery stores.

Most grocery stores have similar layouts; fresh produce, meat, and dairy typically sit along the outer walls while all the fake food populates the middle aisles. As I began to eat healthy, whole foods, I noticed that my grocery store shopping routes changed dramatically. I no longer walked up and down each aisle, examining all the new boxed food products. Instead, I stuck to the outer loop of the store, where you find the real food.

Refined foods not only lack the natural micronutrients found only in whole foods, but they also contain a slew of toxic ingredients. Let's examine some of the toxins masquerading as food, shall we?

I have a weakness for burgers and fries - the quintessential modern American meal. On occasion, I still treat myself to a burger and fries, but I try to make the meal myself using ground turkey (and sometimes organic grass-fed beef) along with sweet potato fries roasted in the oven. However, even this healthier version of a burger and fries is a special treat for me these days. I try to stick to my plant-based whole food diet. Thankfully, I am losing my taste for fast food.

I have neither the time nor the space to cover all the ill effects of fast food in this book. (If you have any doubts, just watch the documentary Super Size Me.) I would, however, like to mention one prevalent toxin: acrylamide.

Classified as a probable carcinogen by the American Cancer Society, acrylamide is a chemical compound that has been used in industrial processes for several decades. But nobody knew that we were eating acrylamide until 2002, when Swedish scientists discovered that high-temperature cooking methods produce acrylamide in food, especially starchy food.

French fries and potato chips are loaded with acrylamide. Acrylamide can form on meat cooked at high temperatures, too. Cooking a well-done steak on a barbecue grill probably isn't a good idea. Low-temperature cooking methods like steaming and boiling are safer. I try to eat raw food for about 50 percent of my diet, and I rarely eat burgers, fries, or chips because they are high in toxins and fats and low in nutrients.

Many (dare I say most) food additives and preservatives are also toxic. A 2007 study at the University of Southampton in the U.K. showed that artificial colors and preservatives can dramatically alter the behavior of children. Participants in the double-blind study who consumed a mix of food coloring and sodium benzoate (a preservative commonly used in sodas) became hyperactive, impulsive, and distracted. Sound familiar? Could it be that sodas, candies, and processed foods are behind the epidemic of attention-deficit hyperactivity disorder (ADHD)?

Professor Jim Stevenson, lead author of the study, wrote that it provided "clear evidence that mixtures of certain food colours and benzoate preservative can adversely influence the behavior of children."

Tartrazine, also known as FD&C Yellow 5, gives macaroni and cheese its bright orange color. It also causes irritability, restlessness, and insomnia among children, according to a study published in the Australian Paediatric Journal. By the way, most FD&C food colorings are made from coal tar. Yum.

I've already mentioned the dangers associated with aspartame. Because of its associated health risks, it took more than a decade for the FDA to approve it. For a detailed disclosure of the shocking political maneuvers behind the approval of aspartame, check out Robyn O'Brien's book The Unhealthy Truth. O'Brien, a mother of four who began investigating the food industry after her daughter had a severe allergic reaction, also brings up serious concerns about genetically modified food.

Genetically modified food first hit the shelves when the FDA approved rBGH milk in 1993. The acronym stands for "recombinant bovine growth hormone." Without getting too technical, rBGH is a genetically engineered hormone made from cow DNA combined with DNA from E. Coli bacteria. This synthetic hormone causes cows to produce more milk, but it turns out that the fake hormone can increase the risk of breast cancer and other types of cancers among humans.

The synthetic hormone harms cows, too. As O'Brien points out, the rBGH package warns of problems like "increases in cystic ovaries and disorder of the uterus" and "increased risk of clinical mastitis." Mastitis is an infection in the cow's udder. Sometimes, the mastitis goes unnoticed and untreated, and the infected cow's inflamed udders squirt out bacteria and pus along with milk. Mmm. I'm sure that concoction does a body good.

I told you this was the Scary Chapter!

When it's noticed, the mastitis is treated with antibiotics and other medications that can end up in your cereal bowl - unless you buy organic milk, that is. As more people learn about rBGH, organic milk is becoming more popular.

Genetically modified corn, on the other hand, is more popular than ever. Most people don't even realize that they're eating so much genetically modified (GM) corn, but 80 percent of the corn grown in the United States is GM corn. GM corn contains a strand of bacterial DNA that causes the corn plant itself to produce a pesticide. GM corn has been shown to cause liver and kidney toxicity as well as hormonal disruption among laboratory rats.

As our nation's largest crop, corn is ubiquitous in refined foods. It's hard to find a condiment or salad dressing that doesn't list high-fructose corn syrup (HFCS) as an ingredient. Even most breads are made with HFCS. Read the ingredients next time you're in the grocery store.

Other GM corn-derived ingredients may include artificial flavorings, artificial sweeteners, baking powder, calcium stearate, caramel, cellulose, dextrose, food starch, gluten, glycerides, hydrolyzed vegetable protein, iodized salt, lysine, malic acid, malt, maltodextrin, maltose, modified food starch, monosodium glutamate (MSG), saccharin, vanillin, xantham gum, and xylitol. Whew - that's a lot of corn! And the above list of corn-derived ingredients is only partial.

By analyzing the molecular structure of hamburgers, one group of researchers found that ninety-three percent of the tissue in a typical fast food burger is derived from corn. That's not too surprising considering that most farmers feed cows a steady diet of corn.

Cows, like humans, are designed to eat nutrient-dense foods like grasses rather than GM corn. A steady diet of corn makes cows more susceptible to illness, which increases the amount of antibiotics in beef and dairy products. Corn-fed beef also contains fifteen to fifty percent less omega-3 fats. If you must eat beef, opt for free-range, grass-fed organic beef.

Even soy, often touted as a health food, can be toxic in excess quantities. Remember, everything in moderation. Vegetarians who consume a lot of soy may be at risk. The isoflavones in soy mimic estrogen, and they're potentially toxic to the thyroid gland. Other toxins in soy may interfere with digestion and absorption of essential minerals.

Like corn, soy is in a wide range of processed foods, from margarine to health foods - and ninety-two percent of the soy grown in the U.S. is genetically modified. In The Unhealthy Truth, O'Brien argues that the new proteins present in genetically modified soy likely played a role in the doubling of child peanut allergy between 1997 and 2002. GM soy was introduced into the U.S. food supply in 1996. It turns out that some of the new proteins in GM soy are similar to peanut proteins responsible for allergic reactions.

We don't know what the long-term effects of GM foods will be. A 2004 study showed that the bacterial DNA in GM soy can be transferred to the bacteria living in the human intestine. The bacteria living in our intestines play an important role in digestion and immune system function. We simply don't know what GM foods might do to our internal environment or our external environment.

GM foods currently on the market include soy, corn, milk, canola, Hawaiian papaya, alfalfa, zucchini, yellow squash, and cotton. (You may be thinking, "Hey, cotton's not a food!" – but cottonseed oil is an ingredient in many processed foods.)

Since GM foods are not labeled, the only way to avoid them is to buy organic. Organic food is grown without the use of genetically modified organisms, pesticides, herbicides, or chemical fertilizers. Of course, you also have to avoid all processed food if you don't want to take your chances with genetically engineered ingredients. Luckily for us, processed foods have low nutrient densities.

We live in a thoroughly toxic world. It's impossible to avoid environmental toxins. Toxins from the products we use, the air we breathe, the water we drink, and the food we eat are killing us. They generate free radicals, promote aging and inflammation, and wear down the immune system. A steady diet of toxins will overwhelm the liver, the body's main organ of detoxification. A liver supports healthy immune system function. When your body becomes toxic, a cleanse is necessary to restore health. A cleanse gives your body a chance to let go of excess toxins. I'll discuss detoxification and cleansing in more detail in Chapter 5.

"Food is the number one cause of illness across the world," says Dr. Michael Lam, MD. "Improper food is accountable for more deaths (due to cancer, diabetes, and heart attacks) than World Wars I and II combined. If food is not toxic, what is?"

Indeed, countless studies show that calorie restriction increases longevity. Mice that eat less live longer. The same seems to hold true for humans. Skinny people live longer. Think about it. As Dr. Lam says, "Have you seen a grossly obese person live to the ripe old age of 100?"

I haven't. But I've seen a lot of people die because they were addicted to toxic food.

Have I scared you sufficiently enough to know that we have a serious dilemma with regard to toxins?

3

The Obesity Epidemic

Jenny was a star athlete in high school. At 120 pounds, she had long, muscular legs and ripped abdominal muscles. Just a few years ago, Jenny excelled at tennis and earned an athletic scholarship to a major university. Today, she looks at an old photo of herself as if it portrays a stranger.

During her second year of college, Jenny sustained an ankle injury that forced her to quit playing tennis. Now in her late 20s, she is more than 100 pounds overweight - medically obese. She suffers from high blood pressure, low back pain, diabetes, depression, and asthma.

"When I played tennis, I exercised every day and watched what I ate. When I got hurt, it's like I totally gave up," Jenny says as tears stream down her plump cheek. "I felt like I had no reason to be healthy anymore. I stopped exercising and started eating whatever I wanted, whenever I wanted. Eating became my sport."

Jenny's honesty and insight and rare. Many people don't realize or admit that they have a problem with overeating. Jenny might have continued down the same dangerous path had she not realized that her 10-year high school reunion is coming up soon. She's determined to lose weight, and she came to me for help.

She didn't come see me because she has early signs of heart disease, American's number one killer. She didn't come see me to get her diabetes under control or even to relieve her back pain. She came to see me because she wants to look good in front of her old high school friends. I'm just glad that she came to see me. Weight loss got her in the door, but now that she's a patient, I can help Jenny overcome the chronic illnesses that are killing her.

All of Jenny's medical problems, even her asthma, stem from her obesity. As Jenny loses weight, her asthma symptoms will improve.

How does obesity affect asthma? you may be wondering. Researchers don't understand all of the mechanisms at this point, but it's clear that being overweight increases the risk and the severity of asthma.

On the simplest level, the mechanics of obesity make it harder to breathe. As you gain weight, fat tissue builds up around internal organs as well as external muscles. The increased pressure from fat tissue can decrease lung capacity, making it more difficult to breathe. On a more complicated level that's not yet fully understood, fat tissue emits inflammatory hormones.

Asthma is an inflammatory disease in which airway muscles tighten. Constricted airways cause asthma attacks. Asthmatics liken attacks to an immense pressure on the chest that's preventing normal breathing. Severe asthma attacks can be fatal. Asthma kills approximately 5,000 Americans each year.

The majority of asthma attacks are triggered by environmental allergens; however, in some cases, the only trigger is systemic inflammation. Remember, fat is not just an inactive blob of tissue. It actively sends out hormones that affect the entire body.

Leptin, for example, is a hormone that plays a major

role in controlling appetite and promoting inflammation. It is an adipokine, a hormone produced by fat tissue. Fat tissue secretes leptin, which increases metabolism and decreases appetite. Leptin has the job of promoting weight loss, but obese individuals who have a habit of eating even when they're not hungry often suffer from leptin resistance. Because the leptin is not doing its job, fat tissue produces more leptin, which can create a constant level of systemic inflammation. As more leptin is secreted into the bloodstream, leptin resistance can increase, causing the formation of even more fat tissue. It's a vicious cycle. Inflammatory adipokines like leptin are associated with asthma as well as atherosclerosis and type II diabetes mellitus.

It's no surprise, then, that Jenny also suffers from diabetes. Type II diabetes, also known as adult-onset diabetes, is caused by insulin resistance. Insulin is another hormone (produced in the pancreas) that helps the body use glucose for energy. After you eat a meal, your blood sugar rises, and insulin signals your cells to take up the glucose in your blood. Overeating combined with a sedentary lifestyle can lead to insulin resistance, in which cells no longer respond to insulin. Therefore, the body produces even more insulin, which makes the insulin resistance worse. Approximately 55 percent of people with Type II diabetes are medically obese. Nearly 90 percent of those with Type II diabetes are overweight.

These days, the obesity epidemic in our modern society is causing many children to develop "adult-onset" diabetes. Environmental toxins may play a role in childhood diabetes, too. For example, increased levels of BPA, that ubiquitous toxin from plastic products, are associated with type II diabetes.

According to the American Diabetes Association, uncontrolled diabetes can lead to heart disease, stroke, high blood pressure, blindness, kidney disease, nervous system damage, amputations, dental disease, pregnancy complications, sexual dysfunction, and other complications.

The good news is that type II diabetes can be kept under control with regular exercise and a healthy diet. The bad news, of course, is that many obese individuals have a hard time changing their lifestyle.

Not even 30-years-old, Jenny also suffers from atherosclerosis and high blood pressure. If she doesn't change her ways soon, she'll develop heart disease at an early age.

Just a few years ago, high cholesterol was thought to be the culprit behind heart disease. Well, that's not quite the case. Now we know that there are different types of cholesterol: High density lipoprotein (HDL) cholesterol is considered "good" while low density lipoprotein (LDL) cholesterol is considered "bad."

Cholesterol is a type of fat that does not dissolve in blood. Everybody needs cholesterol; it is a major component of cell walls, and it helps the body synthesize hormones and vitamin D. Cholesterol becomes problematic when LDL cholesterol sticks to the walls of blood vessels, forming a plaque that narrows the arteries.

HDL cholesterol doesn't stick to arterial walls. It remains in liquid form. In fact, HDL cholesterol can sometimes dislodge solidified LDL cholesterol that's stuck to arterial walls; that's why it's known as the "good" cholesterol.

LDL cholesterol, on the other hand, can build up on the sides of blood vessels. This plaque not only narrows arteries and increases blood pressure, but it also promotes inflammation. The immune system sees the plaque as a foreign substance and attacks it. Over time, such inflammation can damage arteries and cause them to burst. This can lead to blood clots, blockage of arteries, and heart attacks.

Junk food puts one at risk for heart disease by increasing LDL cholesterol. Saturated fats, trans fats, and deep fried foods increase LDL cholesterol. A high-fiber diet can decrease LDL cholesterol. Omega-3 fatty acids, found in flaxseed and cold water fish like salmon, can decrease LDL and increase HDL.

Even eggs (eaten in moderation) can help to decrease LDL cholesterol. Several years ago, doctors advised patients with high cholesterol to avoid eggs. Now we know that eggs, while high in cholesterol, can actually lower the level of bad cholesterol in the body. Eggs contain choline, a component of lecithin, which dissolves cholesterol. Eggs are also a rich source of vitamins and proteins. Eating an egg a day won't kill you. Just make sure that plant foods constitute your main source of nutrients.

Considering all of her health problems, it's clear that Jenny suffers from metabolic syndrome, also known as syndrome X. Metabolic syndrome is a general term that refers to a cluster of risks associated with obesity. In Jenny's case, her obesity and inactive lifestyle put her at high risk for diabetes and heart disease. Signs of metabolic syndrome include type II diabetes, high blood pressure, obesity, low HDL cholesterol, and elevated triglycerides. (Triglycerides are the main constituents of vegetable oils and animal fats, and they're the main components of LDL cholesterol.) A 2002 study estimated that 25 percent of Americans suffer from metabolic syndrome. Many of these individuals will experience diabetes, heart attacks, and strokes.

Jenny's obesity also causes chronic low back pain. The spine supports the body's weight, and excess weight can interfere with spinal alignment.

The lumbar spine, the low back, is particularly susceptible to injury from excess weight. Abdominal fat pulls the body forward and strains the back muscles. The technical term for this exaggerated curve of the spine is lordosis. Obesity can also lead to osteoarthritis, sciatica, herniated disks, degenerative disk disease, and other painful conditions. Low back pain is the leading cause of disability in the United States. I see it every day in my chiropractic clinic. Losing just 10 pounds of excess fat can significantly improve back pain.

When the spinal alignment is compromised in one

area, it usually leads to overcompensation in another part of the spine. For example, my obese patients with low back pain often suffer from neck or shoulder pain as well. A misaligned spine can cause other health problems, too.

A vertebral subluxation occurs when a bone in the spine moves out of its natural position and puts pressure on spinal nerves. Subluxations can cause pain as well as imbalances in neurotransmitters and hormones. Chiropractors perform adjustments to correct subluxations. However, unless the patient loses weight and eradicates the underlying health problem, subluxations will continue to arise.

As we age, gravity becomes a more formidable enemy. Gravity constantly pulls on the body. When we hit middle age, body parts begin to droop and sag. It's not pretty sight, but it's a fact of life. Excess weight multiplies the force of gravity and speeds up aging. Losing weight will help you age more gracefully.

Now, back to Jenny: she also suffers from depression. Obesity can cause anxiety and depression on a social level (ask any Fat Boy), but it can also cause depression on a biochemical level. In Food Addiction, former food addict Kay Sheppard, MA, explains: "Gummy bears and marshmallow chicks can be vicious killers whose effects can lead to depression, irritability, and even suicide. The terrible truth is that for certain individuals, refined carbohydrates can trigger the addictive process."

Refined sugar, Sheppard explains, is an addictive chemical with no nutritional value. When it's consumed, it elevates insulin levels, which in turn elevates endorphin levels. Endorphins are "feel-good" chemicals, but continuous, excessive consumption of refined carbohydrates will cause the body to scale back its own production of endorphins. When the body stops making its own feel-good chemicals, depression sets in. The body then craves more sugar in an effort to restore endorphins. Thus begins the vicious cycle of overeating and food addiction. To avoid this cycle, you have to avoid refined sugar and processed foods; you have to eat whole foods and complex carbohydrates found in fruits and vegetables. We'll discuss food addiction in more detail in the next chapter.

The typical American diet is also high in omega-6 fatty acids (found in vegetable oils and processed foods) and low in omega-3 fatty acids (found in nuts, seeds, and cold-water fish). In 2004, Prevention magazine reported that six out of ten people suffering depression found relief by taking fish oil supplements rich in omega-3 fats, according to a study published in the American Journal of Psychiatry.

"The results were huge, and the improvements were obvious," said Psychiatrist Andrew Stoll, MD, of Harvard Medical School. "Those who got the supplements slept better and felt less worthlessness and guilt. We think omega-3s help your brain use a feel-good chemical called serotonin."

Food allergies can cause depression, too. There are different types of food allergies, and not all of them cause immediate reactions. You may be sensitive to certain foods without even knowing it. Delayed food allergies, or food sensitivities, are often difficult to detect, but they can have a devastating impact on your mood. For instance, many people have sensitivities to casein (milk protein) and gluten (wheat protein). Eating foods to which you are sensitive can cause mood changes as well as other symptoms such as fatigue, headaches, and digestive problems. A simple blood test will let you know which foods, if any, you should avoid.

More often than not, it's the food that you eat all the time that's causing an adverse reaction. If you eat a lot of dairy or wheat, try avoiding the food completely for two weeks. (Be sure to avoid all the dairy or wheat in processed foods, too!) Then slowly reintroduce the food to your diet and see what happens. You may be surprised to learn that your favorite food is actually your worst enemy.

Heavy metals in your food may also cause depression. In our toxic world, large fish like tuna and swordfish typically contain high levels of mercury. Earlier this year, researchers discovered that nearly half of commercial samples of high-fructose corn syrup (HFCS) contain mercury. HFCS, as I pointed out in the last chapter, is in everything from soda to bread. When heavy metals like mercury build up in your body, they can affect your immune, endocrine, neurological, and cardiovascular systems. Our food has become an industrial product, contaminated with industrial chemicals.

If you're eating a diet of processed foods, you're not getting enough nutrients, and that can affect your state of mind, too. Vitamin deficiency, for instance, can cause depression. As Psychology Today reported in 2004, "Fatigue, irritability, poor concentration, anxiety and depression - all can be signs of a B vitamin deficiency." Refined food destroys B vitamins; alcohol, nicotine, and caffeine also destroy B vitamins. Good dietary sources of B vitamins include dark leafy greens, sea vegetables, nuts, and fish.

Vitamin D deficiency can cause depression as well. Our skin produces vitamin D from sunlight, but unless you sunbathe for 30 minutes at high noon every day, you're probably not getting enough vitamin D. I recommend a quality vitamin D supplement to all of my patients.

A recent study found that two out of five small children have less than optimal levels of vitamin D. If you have children, encourage them to go outdoors and play as much as possible.

Mineral deficiencies can cause depression, anxiety, and sleep disorders. Several studies have concluded that the typical American diet is lacking in magnesium. Stress further depletes magnesium. A magnesium deficiency can cause confusion, agitation, and depression, as well as physical problems. Dark green leafy vegetables and pumpkin seeds are rich sources of magnesium.

Finally, refined foods can cause depression and other health problems by disrupting the balance of microorganisms in your gut. Fungal and bacterial organisms live in our gut. Normally, the good bacteria keep the bad microbes at bay; however, if you kill off a substantial number of the good bacteria, harmful organisms can take over.

Candida are yeast-like fungal organisms that are normally present in the digestive system. For most people, candida are harmless. But sometimes, usually because of poor diet or use of certain medications, candida can grow out of control, causing a condition called candidiasis.

Refined sugars and processed foods feed candida and bad bacteria, whereas good bacteria prefer whole fruits and vegetables. If you're not eating a healthy diet, or if you use antibiotics without restoring healthy bacteria (probiotics), candidiasis can set in. Candida produce toxic byproducts that end up in the bloodstream, where they may affect the brain and cause depression. Candida overgrowth may also reduce magnesium absorption in the intestine, which can also lead to depression. Signs of candidiasis include oral thrush, white patches inside the cheeks, and frequent yeast infections.

Severe candidiasis can lead to leaky gut syndrome, in which the organisms bore holes in the intestinal walls. The holes allow food particles to leak into parts of the body where they shouldn't be. Leaky gut syndrome often results in severe food sensitivities, as the immune system begins to attack those stray food particles as if they're foreign invaders. A detox diet – or a candida cleanse – can restore a healthy balance to intestinal flora by starving the candida and allowing good bacteria to grow.

A poor diet can cause depression through several different mechanisms. If you eat a whole food diet and avoid refined food, you'll greatly diminish your chances of suffering from depression.

As an obese young woman, Jenny faces another health challenge that's not so apparent: an increased risk of developing cancer. Hundreds of studies show that obesity increases the risk of common cancers like breast cancer and kidney cancer as well as less common cancers like leukemia and melanoma.

Excess fat promotes inflammation, and inflammation promotes cancer. A 2007 study in the journal Cell reported a possible mechanism by which chronic inflammation may cause cancer.

"Although there is plenty of evidence that chronic inflammation can promote cancer, the cause of this relationship is not understood," said Alexander Hoffmann, assistant professor of chemistry and biochemistry at U.C. San Diego, who led the study. "We have identified a basic cellular mechanism that we think may be linking chronic inflammation and cancer."

A protein known as p100 facilitates communication between the inflammatory and cellular development processes. Some amount of communication is beneficial, but too much communication (which results from chronic inflammation) can lead to unrestrained cell development (cancer).

"Studies with animals have shown that a little inflammation is necessary for the normal development of the immune system and other organ systems," said Hoffmann. "We discovered that the protein p100 provides the cell with a way in which inflammation can influence development. But there can be too much of a good thing. In the case of chronic inflammation, the presence of too much p100 may over activate the developmental pathway, resulting in cancer."

Indeed, obesity may account for 30 percent of several major cancers, including cancers of the colon, breast, kidney, and esophagus. Regular exercise combined with a healthy diet will lower your risk of cancer. One study found that women who intentionally lost 20 pounds, down to a healthy weight, decreased their cancer rates to the level of healthy women who were never overweight.

Heart disease is the number one killer of Americans, and cancer comes in a close second. If you're obese, your chance of dying from heart disease or cancer is very high – unless you lose weight and keep it off.

Are You Obese?

Obesity is a medical condition in which excess fat adversely affects health and shortens lifespan. The National Heart Lung and Blood Institute (NHLBI) defines obese individuals as those with a Body Mass Index (BMI) of 30 or higher.

You can calculate your BMI using a simple mathematical formula. It's based on a ratio of weight to height. To calculate your BMI, measure your height in inches and weight in pounds. Multiply your weight by 703. Divide the result by your height, then take that result and divide it by your height again.

For example, I'm 6'1" (73 inches) and weigh 210 pounds. Here's how I calculate my BMI:

$$210 \times 703 = 147630$$
$$147630 / 73 = 2022.3$$
$$2022.3 / 73 = 27.7$$

With a BMI of 27.7, I'm considered overweight but not obese. At 5'4" and 225 pounds, Jenny currently has a BMI of 38.6, which is considered medically obese.

Here's the standard BMI classification system from the NHLBI:

Underweight = 18.5 or less

Normal weight = 18.5 to 24.9

Overweight = 25 to 29.9

Obese = BMI of 30 or greater

As your BMI increases, your lifespan decreases. A BMI of 30 to 35 reduces life expectancy by two to four years. A BMI of 40 or greater reduces life expectancy by 20 years for men and five years for women. Just think: You may be able to add 20 years to your life by losing weight! I know that weight loss is difficult, but I'm living proof that it's possible.

With a BMI of 27.7, I'm still overweight, and I'm still working to get down to a healthy weight. One thing I've learned over the years is that the more weight you lose, the harder it is to lose weight, but I'm still steadily dropping the pounds, and I feel better than I have in years.

Tracking the Obesity Epidemic

According to the Centers for Disease Control and Prevention (CDC), thirty-four percent of U.S. adults are obese, and nearly seventy percent of Americans are overweight. Numbering 72 million, obese Americans outnumber the total population of France. In 1980, only fifteen percent of Americans were obese.

What has changed since 1980? Our environment and our food supply have become more toxic. Cheap, processed foods that are high in calories and low in nutrition have become staples of the American diet. The industrialization of the food industry has polluted our food supply.

A hundred years ago, poor people were typically skinnier than those who were wealthy. Now, that trend is reversed. Cheap, processed food is readily available even to those who don't have much money. In fact, in most cases, poor people must buy more processed food to live within their means. A single mother making minimum wage cannot afford to buy organic, whole foods. Sadly, it's just not feasible, and this is reflected in the CDC statistics. For instance, fifty-three percent of black women and 51 percent of Mexican-American women aged 40 to 59 are obese, compared to thirty-nine percent of white women in the same age group. Socioeconomic status accounts for these disparities.

Unfortunately, I don't see this trend changing until our healthcare system changes. In Europe, for instance, many food manufacturers have removed harmful additives from their food. Yet, in the U.S., the same manufacturers keep those ingredients in our food. Why?

Is it possible in Europe, tax payer dollars fund healthcare. That creates a common interest in everyone's healthcare. When somebody gets sick, everybody has to pay for it; therefore, the society as a whole demands a universal supply of healthy, nutritious food. In America, who cares if Joe Blow is eating toxic soup? That's his business, right? After all, we won't have to pay for his cardiac bypass surgery. Until that fundamental attitude changes, toxic food will continue to corrupt our food supply.

Fat: It's Not All Bad

Some amount of body fat is necessary. Fat not only provides padding to protect our internal organs, but it also protects us from toxic chemicals. When your liver cannot process all the toxins coming into your body, excess toxins get stored in fat tissue (and some toxins get stored in the liver itself).

If you're carrying around excess fat, on the other hand, that means you're also carrying around more toxins. As fat cells get burned for energy, toxins are released into your bloodstream. The cycle of yo-yo dieting results in maximum exposure to toxins. When you keep losing and regaining weight, you're releasing a never-ending stream of toxins into your body. Give your liver a break!

In order to lose weight, keep it off, and minimize your exposure to toxins, you need to do your best to avoid harmful chemicals (in processed foods and other environmental toxins), and you need to regularly detoxify your body.

In Chapter 5, you'll learn how to safely cleanse your body of toxins. Once you get rid of the toxins, it will be easier for you to lose weight and keep it off. Your body can then devote more energy to burning fat and protecting you from disease rather than processing toxins.

Whether you want to increase your longevity or look good for your high school reunion, you can break the cycle of yo-yo dieting once and for all.

4

Food Addiction

Several years ago, a good friend of mine named Don came to see me because of his back pain. A specialist had suggested back surgery, and Don wisely decided to consult with me before submitting to surgery. Together we outlined an exercise and stretching program, and Don's back started feeling better. He was able to avoid that surgery.

But there was another problem: Don needed to lose about 100 pounds. He knew he was overweight, but he didn't come to me to lose weight. I don't think he really wanted to lose weight. He was addicted to food.

So I started talking to him about the importance of losing weight, extinguishing the flames of inflammation, and getting his blood pressure under control. I outlined a plan for weight loss. Always an optimist, Don said, "Yeah, I'm gonna do that, doc. I'm gonna lose weight and get healthy."

When he came in the next month, Don had actually gained weight.

"What happened?" I asked him.

"It's just too hard, doc," he said with uncharacteristic pessimism. "I just can't do it. We go out to eat with all our friends several times a week, and we eat and talk. That's what we do, and it's my favorite thing to do. I just can't lose the weight. It's too hard."

When I went home that night, I told my son about Don's situation.

"I just don't understand," I told him. "He's going to die if he doesn't lose weight, and the fear of death won't get him to change his eating habits. He says it's too hard."

My son is a healthy young man with his head square on his shoulders. He thought for a moment and said, "Is it harder than dying? Because that's what's gonna happen if he doesn't change."

"I know," I said.

So I tried a different approach with Don. I waited for him to tell me that weight loss is too hard.

"Is it harder than dying?" I asked, raising my voice a little. "Is it harder than what you're going to put your family through when you're lying there in the hospital with heart disease, close to death, with your family around you, knowing that you've let them all down?"

Don thought about what I said, and something seemed to click.

"Doc, you're right," he said. "You got me motivated. I'm gonna do it. I'm gonna lose the weight."

When Don came back the next month, he had gained weight again. He was beginning to show signs of severe illness.

"We've got to get this weight off you somehow," I said to my friend.

"I just can't do it," he replied. "It's too hard."

It wasn't long before Don was having the symptoms of a heart attack. They were minor symptoms, mind you – clamminess, chest pains, pain down the left arm – but I knew something wasn't right. I asked Don to call his medical doctor and tell him that his friend Dr. Doug thought he was having a heart attack.

His doctor must've been some diagnostician; he didn't even need to see Don to tell him: "Aw, I don't think you're having a heart attack. Just take a couple of aspirins. Your friend's a chiropractor. He doesn't know what he's talking about."

That was good enough for Don. He didn't want to admit

that he might have heart disease. So I did what any good friend would do: I convinced his wife to take him to a clinic.

"Take him right now," I told her.

She did, and they ended up rushing Don to the hospital. He was having a heart attack.

I went to visit him in the hospital, and he didn't even mention his weight. His back pain had returned, and he wanted me to help him with that. I continued to visit him in the hospital to perform adjustments and massages, but his back pain just kept getting worse.

"Don, we've got to do something about your lifestyle," I finally said. "You're not going to get better until you make some changes. You've got to lose some weight and starting eating proper nutrition."

"I want to, doc, I really do, but I just can't do it, and I don't know why," he said.

At that point, it seemed as if he had lost his optimistic attitude and given up all hope. Don was never able to make the changes necessary to save his life. He passed away.

Don's death provided the answer to my son's question:

Is losing weight harder than dying? YES!

For many food addicts, losing weight is harder than dying - just as many alcoholics find it easier to die than to put down the bottle.

But, for you and me it's not too late.

Indeed, the similarities between food addiction and alcoholism (or any drug addiction) are striking. On a fundamental neurochemical level, there's not much difference.

Food addiction and drug addiction share the same neural pathway: the mesolimbic dopamine system. This pathway in the midbrain controls our reward and reinforcement behaviors. Dopamine, like serotonin, is a feel-good chemical. Whenever you have sex, eat, or ingest certain mind-altering substances (like coffee, for instance, or crack cocaine), your brain releases dopamine as a reward. This neurochemical reward reinforces the behavior, prompting you to seek out that good feeling again in the future.

The midbrain is a primal part of the brain that hasn't quite caught up to modern times. Several hundred years ago, the midbrain worked well to promote the survival of our species. Sex, for instance, obviously promotes the survival of the species. Therefore, whenever you have sex, your midbrain gives you a little neurochemical cookie. But in our modern society, sex has become a commodity as well as a means of reproduction. It's just a phone call or a click away. The National Council on Sexual Addiction Compulsivity estimates that up to 24 million Americans are addicted to sex.

The midbrain also releases dopamine after you eat. Eating, like sex, is necessary for the survival of the species. But, like sex, food has become a commodity rather than simply a source of energy. Food is now a product, and the largest food manufacturers spend millions of dollars to create an emotional connection between you and their product.

Last night I saw a TV commercial full of happy, skinny people stuffing their faces with burgers and fries. I won't lie; for a split second, the commercial stimulated my midbrain, and felt a craving for a burger. Fortunately, my forebrain knew better.

In days of yore, the midbrain rewarded overeating, too. Back then, the midbrain never knew when a famine might strike, so it rewarded people for storing up extra energy in the form of fat tissue. Those people with extra reserves of energy had a better chance of survival. Today, in our society, the famine never comes, yet food addicts keep packing on the pounds.

"They do not eat to survive. They love eating and spend the day planning their new takeout choices," said Mark Gold, M.D., chief of addiction medicine at the McKnight Brain Institute at the University of Florida, after studying "people who were too heavy to leave their reclining chairs and too big to walk out the doorway."

Another reason that overeating is so common in our society is because people aren't getting enough nutrition. The most popular foods - pizza, pasta, burgers, fries, etc. - are low in nutrients and high in calories. When you're not getting enough nutrients, your brain tells you to eat more. But if you continue to eat low-nutrient, high-calorie foods, you'll simply gain weight without getting the benefits of proper nutrition. That's why it's so important to eat a plant-based diet that will provide your body with all the nutrients it needs.

Think about how a car works. To keep a car running properly, you can't just keep filling it up with fuel, and you can't give it too much fuel or the tank will overflow. You could conceivably give it more fuel by adding extra gas tanks, but eventually the car would become too bulky, and its performance would suffer. To keep a vehicle running properly, you have to give it the right amount of gas, change its oil, replace the antifreeze, adjust the suspension, etc. Similarly, you have to supply your body with vitamins, minerals, and phytonutrients as well as energy yielding nutrients (fats, carbs and protein). And you have to keep your suspension working well, too!

The primitive midbrain is not very smart. It doesn't know the difference between energy-providing macronutrients and other necessary micronutrients. If you're not eating proper nutrition, your midbrain will tell you to have another slice of pizza, even though that pizza is providing the equivalent of gasoline when your body really needs antifreeze. (Note: Do not eat antifreeze. No part of your brain will reward that behavior.)

I've found that people can become addicted to either high-fat foods or high-sugar foods - but the most addictive foods are those with high levels of both refined sugars and refined fats. Fast food, pizza, doughnuts, cinnamon rolls, ice cream – these are the kind of foods that fuel addiction. Dr. Gold of the McKnight Brain Institute suggests that these types of foods trigger a larger release of dopamine: "It may be that doughnuts with high fat and high sugar cause more brain reward than soup."

Interestingly, one study found that sweet, high-fat foods are preferred by those with binge-eating disorders, while anorexics tend to have an aversion to fat.

In The End of Overeating, Dr. David Kessler, former commissioner of the FDA, argues that people may become addicted to high-salt foods as well as high-sugar and high-fat foods. Each time one of these foods of desire is consumed by a food addict, the brain releases dopamine.

Keep in mind that Dr. Kessler is the former head of the FDA! In his book, he reveals that food manufacturers intentionally engineer foods that are likely to trigger overeating and food addiction. Food manufacturers and restaurants strive to find the perfect balance of sugar, fat, and salt known as the "bliss point."

"Simply put, American processed food is 'food crack,'" writes Dr. Tom Robinson, MD, in America's Food Addiction. "Crack cocaine is an extremely concentrated form of cocaine that is designed to get the user addicted on the first use. American food chemistry has made processed food taste so intense, the user will be tempted to overeat themselves into poor health and even death. American foods are specifically designed to sell and to keep the customer coming back. Nutritional value is not a consideration, unless a nutritional claim is part of that product's marketing strategy or unless an FDA minimum nutrition requirement is involved."

"American food chemistry is made worse by the fact that many nutritional elements of food (vitamins, minerals, fiber, etc) are removed in the processing," continues Dr. Robinson. "We eat food that tastes great but is high in calories and provides little use as the fuel our bodies need to make us healthy people. As a result, we spend much of our time fatigued, depressed, in pain, and gaining weight."

In 2008, Farai Chideya of National Public Radio interviewed "Vic," a member of Overeaters Anonymous, who described the pain that results from food addiction. On a typical day, Vic would eat several half gallons of ice cream. She felt like she had to keep eating. At night, she would toss and turn because of all the excess food in her stomach. She also experienced night sweats (because her body was trying to eliminate excess toxins). In the morning, she would wake up with a hangover from overeating. Vic described her food hangovers as follows: "My head feels like it's stuffed with concrete cotton. Every nerve in my body feels like it's got acid on it." Vic also felt demoralized, physically ugly, and bloated every morning. That's the life of a food addict. Vic was fortunate. She sought professional help, and she has now recovered from her addiction.

So many processed food ingredients seem to be designed to make you crave food. I don't have time to go over all of them, but I'd like to address three of the most dangerous food additives on the market: HFCS, aspartame, and MSG. All three of these chemicals contribute to the obesity epidemic.

High fructose corn syrup (HFCS), rather than cane sugar, is used to sweeten most processed food. Why? Because it's cheap and plentiful. The government gives out roughly $40 billion (yes, that's billion with a B) in subsidies to corn growers in each year. Corn is the nation's largest crop.

In There is a Cure for Diabetes, Dr. Gabriel Cousens writes, "Corn syrup has been singled out by many health experts as one of the chief culprits of rising obesity, because corn syrup does not turn off appetite. Since the advent of corn syrup, consumption of all sweeteners has soared, as have people's weights. According to a 2004 study reported in the American Journal of Clinical Nutrition, the rise of Type-2 diabetes since 1980 has closely paralleled the increased use of sweeteners, particularly corn syrup."

Andreas Moritz agrees with Dr. Cousens' assessment in Timeless Secrets of Health & Rejuvenation: "Since the fructose in corn syrup does neither stimulate insulin secretion nor reduce the hunger hormone ghrelin, you will continue to feel hungry while the body converts the fructose into fat. The resulting obesity increases the risk of diabetes and other diseases."

A recent study found that HFCS can induce leptin resistance. Leptin, remember, is the hormone that regulates your metabolism and appetite; it signals the body when it's time to stop eating. HFCS is literally altering our biochemistry in a manner that causes us to eat more. HFCS plays a big role in the obesity epidemic - and it's everywhere! Stop drinking soda, and start reading ingredient labels carefully. Even better, avoid all processed food.

While HFCS is refined from corn, aspartame (the sweetener marketed to those of us who are trying to lose weight) is made from scratch in the laboratory. Aspartame is the chemical name for NutraSweet, Equal, and Spoonful. I've already mentioned that aspartame accounts for over 75 percent of adverse reactions to food additives reported to the FDA. And even though it's the low-calorie sweetener, aspartame has been shown to stimulate the appetite, causing food cravings and weight gain.

Mary Nash Stoddard, founder of the Aspartame Consumer Safety Network, said, "It's well documented that excitotoxins like aspartame have the reverse affect on weight. People drinking diet drinks and eating diet food will get more hungry. The FDA no longer allows manufacturers of diet supplement drinks and foods containing aspartame to label them as weight reduction products, but requires that they be labeled as diet drink or diet food. A study of 80,000 women who use sweeteners were evaluated through the Centers for Disease Control. It was found that they gained rather than lost weight using artificial sweeteners."

Aspartame is not the only culprit when it comes to

artificial sweeteners. Splenda has been shown to kill good bacteria in the intestines. Even stevia, the naturally sweet herb that's becoming popular among major food manufacturers, though it is a better choice may cause health problems when consumed in excess.

If you want to lose weight, throw out all that processed diet food made with artificial sweeteners. Eat unrefined foods with high nutrient densities, and eat plenty of them!

Like aspartame, monosodium glutamate (MSG) is an excitotoxin. Excitotoxins poison brain cells causing them to over-stimulate. This over-stimulation likely contributes to hyperactivity disorders.

In the public eye, MSG has become associated with Chinese food over the years. It is indeed used as a flavor enhancer in Chinese food (and many Chinese restaurants now market their food as "MSG-free"), but today MSG is in all sorts of processed food. It is commonly found in baby food, fast food, food from chain restaurants, canned food, and frozen food.

In his book In Bad Taste: The MSG Symptom Complex, Dr. George Schwartz, M.D., explains that MSG is an addictive, toxic drug that's added to food. It contributes to obesity, overeating, ADHD, and several neurodegenerative diseases.

"MSG is a drug," explains Dr. Schwartz. "It has no flavor of its own. It synthetically heightens our awareness of food by altering the way the tongue, the nervous system and the brain communicate with each other. It intensifies the flavor of savory foods by causing neuron cells in the mouth to over-react to different flavors. Unfortunately, these over stimulated cells exhaust themselves and die, causing microscopic scarring throughout the human system. Within 30 minutes of eating processed foods high in MSG, neurons swell up like balloons and die after three hours."

MSG is such a powerful drug that researchers all over the world use it to create obese lab rats and mice! MSG triples the amount of insulin produced by the pancreas, so it can quickly lead to insulin resistance and weight gain. Have you ever heard someone say that they feel hungry again just an hour after eating at a Chinese buffet? That's likely because of the MSG in the food.

Here's a partial list of other ingredients that likely contain MSG: Hydrolyzed vegetable protein, Modified enzymes, Barley malt, Calcium caseinate, Maltodextrin, Malt extract, Pectin, Plant protein extract, Sodium caseinate, Textured protein, Yeast extract, Broth, Bullion, and Flavoring or "Natural Flavoring."

Unless you eat a diet consisting of whole, unrefined foods, you cannot avoid MSG. Like HFCS, it's everywhere!

Now that we've covered the basics of food addiction and why food is addictive, let's discuss how to break the addiction.

My whole approach toward dieting changed when I realized that I was addicted to food. I started studying alcoholism and drug addiction as well as organizations like Alcoholics Anonymous, the original 12-step support group. AA has been around since 1935 and currently has over two million members. Obviously, this program helps a lot of people overcome addiction.

I won't go over all 12 steps, but to summarize, they include admitting that you have a problem, taking a personal inventory, gaining spiritual strength through prayer or meditation, and spreading the message of AA.

I have never been to an AA meeting, but I interviewed a friend who is very active in the organization. We'll call him "TJ." TJ has been sober for 19 years, and he gave me valuable insights into the AA recovery program.

The central message of AA is: Don't drink. No matter what happens, don't drink. Unfortunately, I can't tell my weight loss clients: "Don't eat." That just doesn't work. We have to eat! But I can say, "Don't eat junk food. Don't eat refined food. Don't eat toxic food."

A food addict struggles with cravings just as an alcoholic

does. The first step in breaking the addiction is to cleanse the system. Once you flush the toxins from your system, cravings will subside. We'll discuss cleansing in more detail in the next chapter.

Many times, an alcoholic will need to go to an in-house treatment center to detox. Food addicts may need a change in scenery and increased support as well. Health retreats and spas, for example, help many people overcome addictions to junk food.

Luckily, most food addicts can overcome their addictions without going away to a treatment center. But let me warn you: it's tough. The social pressures are enormous.

TJ tells me that during his first month of sobriety, he saw beer ads, beer commercials, and empty beer cans everywhere. I know exactly what he's talking about. Junk food advertisements are just as pervasive.

Even more powerful than advertisements are people. In AA, members tell each other that they must change their "playmates and playgrounds" if they want to succeed in sobriety. My friend Don couldn't do this. He kept going out to eat at the same restaurants and hanging out with the same friends (many of whom were also overeating). Don couldn't change, and he died an early death as a result.

I understand how difficult this type of change can be. Trust me. Our identities get all wrapped up in who we spend time with and what we spend our time doing.

If I were to stop hanging out with my closest group of friends, what would I do? If I were to change my career or give up my favorite relaxation ritual, what would I do? Who would I be? That's the scariest part of change.

The ego loves comfortable routines and fears losing its sense of self. But the egoic mind often behaves like a spoiled child. It craves attention. The good news is that you can transcend the egoic mind. That's where prayer and meditation come into play. Prayer and meditation create a calm, quiet mind that's capable of recognizing a higher power in the universe. When you see that your life has a deeper meaning than your daily routine, it's not as hard to change that routine. We'll discuss spirituality and spiritual cleansing in the next chapter.

Change is difficult and frightening - but life is change. It's better to embrace change and take that unknown leap of faith than to be stuck standing in the same place. A rolling stone gathers no fat.

After a full recovery, food addicts, like alcoholics, may find that they can return to their old playgrounds and playmates without fear of relapse. There's no set time for recovery. The recovery process is different for everybody. Your cravings may disappear after a week, or they may last for years.

Until you have fully recovered from your addiction, you should try to avoid all triggers. For an alcoholic, triggers might include old drinking buddies, certain bars or restaurants, or even certain songs. For a food addict, triggers might include dining buddies, certain restaurants, or certain television programs. For example, if you always ate ice cream when you were watching The Biggest Loser, then you should probably find another show to watch during your recovery. Something as simple as a television show can trigger a craving. Other triggers might be a certain time of day or a certain time of the year. Holidays are notorious for causing relapses among both alcoholics and food addicts.

You can't avoid all triggers. In our society, slick advertisements and merchants are peddling toxic booze and toxic food around every corner. So what should you do when a trigger arises? In AA, they tell newcomers to call a member of the group if they feel the desire to drink. Calling someone interrupts the trigger, and it also provides the alcoholic with social support and a sense of accountability.

Whether you're addicted to carbs or cocaine, accountability is important. That's why I have my patients come into my office for weekly weigh-ins. If they have gained weight, I hold them accountable, and we examine why they gained weight.

When I get a new weight loss patient, we also take a personal inventory. We review all of their problems and their goals. We discuss what has prevented them from achieving their goals in the past and how to overcome those obstacles.

I encourage my patients to seek out other "accountability buddies" and support systems, too. If they're tempted to stray off course, they can call me or one of their buddies. When I went on my first diet as a kid, I lost a lot of weight because I knew I'd have to weigh-in at the next TOPS meeting. I didn't want to have to tell the whole group that I was a pig! Groups like TOPS, Overeaters Anonymous, and Food Addicts Anonymous provide accountability as well as social support. Do a Google search and see which support groups are available in your area.

It helps to be in the company of others who are going through the same thing as you. You can discuss your fears and frustrations and get them off your chest. You can also learn coping techniques that have worked for others.

It also helps to be around people who are concerned about their health. Get a gym membership, take a yoga class, join a softball team, or take up jogging in the park. Find a form of exercise that you'll enjoy. Sometimes, when we get stuck in our daily routines, it may seem as if nobody cares about their health. Why, then, should we? Why can't we have our burger and fries, too? But when you take that leap of faith and venture outside your daily routine, you'll find that plenty of other people care about their health - and when you spend time with such people, you'll begin to care more about your health, too. It's human nature. We're social creatures.

One of the most surprising things that I learned from TJ is that AA puts the responsibility of recovery squarely on the individual who seeks it. If somebody comes into a meeting and says that they want to go out and have a drink after the meeting, the members will often tell that person to go have their drink and enjoy it.

"If you're not ready for recovery, then go back out there and drink some more until you're ready," said TJ, relaying what he told some fellow members of AA. "You'll either end up back here in this room, in jail, in a psych ward, or dead. AA is for the people who want it, not the people who need it."

That's a powerful statement. Think about it for a minute: The support system is for those who want it but not necessarily those who need it. You have to really want to quit drinking before you can take advantage of what AA has to offer.

In the same sense, you have to really want to stop eating junk food to succeed at weight loss. I spend a lot of time with new patients discussing their motivating factors. Surprisingly, the fear of death doesn't seem to be a good motivator.

Several years ago, I told my friend Don that he would die unless he changed his ways. The fear of death didn't motivate him. This was before I started studying food addiction. Today, if Don were still around, I would help him identify other motivating factors.

I don't think Don really wanted to lose weight. He never internalized the desire for weight loss. In Don's case, weight loss was a goal that originated from an external rather than an internal source. He needed to lose weight, but he didn't want it.

In Types of Motivation, Professor Param J. Shah and Ken Shah identify six different types of motivation:

Achievement Motivation: It is the drive to pursue and attain goals. An individual with achievement motivation wishes to achieve objectives and advance up on the ladder of success. Here, accomplishment is important for its own sake and not for the rewards that accompany it.

Affiliation Motivation: It is a drive to relate to people on a social basis. Persons with affiliation motivation perform work better when they are complimented for their favorable attitudes and co-operation.

Competence Motivation: It is the drive to be good at something, allowing the individual to perform high quality work. Competence motivated people seek job mastery, take pride in developing and using their problem-solving skills and strive to be creative when confronted with obstacles. They learn from their experience.

Power Motivation: It is the drive to influence people and change situations. Power motivated people wish to create an impact on their organization and are willing to take risks to do so.

Attitude Motivation: Attitude motivation is how people think and feel. It is their self confidence, their belief in themselves, their attitude to life. It is how they feel about the future and how they react to the past.

Incentive Motivation: It is where a person or a team reaps a reward from an activity. "You do this and you get that."

Fear Motivation: Fear motivation coerces a person to act against will. It is instantaneous and gets the job done quickly. It is helpful in the short run.

Fear motivation may work in the short term, but it rarely lasts. It is a negative motivator. If you have kids, you know that fear only works up to a certain point. The best way to influence a child's behavior is to lead by example; that's a form of positive motivation.

Today, I try to help people discover positive motivating factors that work for them. For instance, Jenny is motivated to lose weight by imagining how good she'll look in her dress at her 10-year high school reunion. I have a feeling that this motivator will work well for her. We'll discuss positive visualization techniques in more detail in Chapter 10.

Different people with different personalities require different motivating factors. What works for some will not work for others. Fear might work for some people, but I can tell you from experience that it doesn't work for most people. I try to help patients discover the simplest motivating factors that will work. The simpler, the better, in my opinion.

Why do you want to lose weight? What is your primary motivating factor?

In a web poll at about.com, 65 percent of participants indicated that they wanted to lose weight to improve their appearance, while only 35 percent indicated that they wanted to lose weight to improve their health.

Fortunately, you don't have to choose one or the other. (That would be a tough decision!) When you lose weight, you will look better, feel better, and enjoy better health.

To discover what motivates you, you must set realistic goals. Many of my patients lose five to ten pounds during their first seven-day cleanse. Some patients lose 20 pounds or more during that first week. When you flush the toxins out of your system, your body will be able to let go of that excess fat.

Some patients don't lose as much weight initially, and that's okay! The more weight you have to lose, the easier it will be in the beginning. For the typical patient who is about 30 pounds overweight, we set an initial weight loss goal of two pounds per week and adjust the goal accordingly.

When you meet your goals, reward yourself. That doesn't mean you should go to the all-you-can-eat Chinese buffet and get extra desert after you lose two pounds, but you should give yourself some type of reward, even if it's something as simple as going to see a movie or buying yourself a new outfit. Using a trial and error approach, you'll find the motivating factors that work best for you.

Conversely, when you gain weight, you must hold yourself accountable. Why did you gain weight? Was it because you skipped a couple of workout sessions? Was it because you went out for lunch a couple of days during the week? You also need a plan that you can put into action as soon as you realize that you've gained weight. When my patients gain weight, they go on a mini-cleanse, and they usually end up losing what they gained plus a couple more pounds.

All of my patients begin their weight loss program with

a seven-day cleanse. The cleanse will allow you to break the cycle of addiction. Again, it won't always be easy. I've seen patients break down in tears during that first week. A few have even lashed out at me in anger.

Remember, when you burn fat cells, the toxins that were bound to those fat cells are released into your body. A cleanse will help your body flush out the toxins, but you may feel the effects of the toxins coursing through your bloodstream. During your initial seven-day cleanse, you may feel nauseated or get headaches at times. That's okay. Your body will soon be rid of the toxins behind your symptoms.

You may also experience withdrawal symptoms during your first cleanse, especially if you normally eat a lot of refined sugar. You may feel fatigued or irritable; you may also experience headaches or nausea. Just remember that these feelings will not last. They are simply signals that your body is adjusting to your new healthy lifestyle. Once you get the toxins out of your system, the symptoms of withdrawal will subside. Have faith. The results are well worth it.

I lost 13 pounds during my first seven-day cleanse, and my triglycerides and blood pressure normalized. But for me, a long-time food addict, the most miraculous benefit of the cleanse was that I no longer craved junk food at the end of the week. I actually enjoyed eating healthy, whole foods. My cravings for pizza transformed into cravings for steamed vegetables. My body was finally getting the nutrients that it needed.

When the going gets tough (and it will), don't give up hope. Instead, use a lifeline and phone a friend. Call up your accountability buddy, your health practitioner, or any positive influence in your life, and talk about your frustrations. Talking about your problems will allow you to continue making the right choice – the healthy choice.

I tell all of my patients that it takes 40 days to make or break a habit. The Christian tradition of Lent, which is a period of fasting or cleansing, lasts for 40 days. The Bible makes several references to 40 days. Jesus fasted for 40 days before he began his ministry. Moses spent 40 days with God on Mount Sinai. And of course, the rain that caused the great flood of Noah's time lasted for 40 days.

Many people agree that it takes 40 days to change a habit. There are two kinds of habits: Good habits and bad habits. You can't change a habit. You can only replace a bad habit with a good habit. In your life, if you have all the habits which are moving you toward good in your life, you will end up with the good habit's rewards. If you have destructive habits, you will always end up as a physical wreck, mentally and emotionally strained, and spiritually defunct.

For example, a bad habit is coming home from work, flopping down on the couch with a beer and the remote control. A good habit would be to come home from work, put on sweat pants and get on my bicycle for 30 minutes or an hour. When you make up your mind to replace a bad habit with a good habit it takes 40 days of consistent, unbroken routine to make it your new reality.

Do you think you can try my weight loss plan for 40 days? When you think about it, 40 days is a short span of time – but so much can happen in 40 days. A seed can grow into a flower in just 40 days. And you – you can reset your body's biochemistry and can change your destiny.

My destiny has certainly changed! After cleansing and detoxing, I not only lost weight and got healthier, but I also felt more alive physically, mentally, and spiritually.

My friend TJ tells me that in AA, they have a saying that goes something like this: "If you want to keep it, you've got to give it away."

TJ says that "it" can refer to serenity as well as sobriety. Sobriety allows an alcoholic to experience serenity, you see. By cleansing and adopting a whole food diet, I was able to experience a serenity of my own. According to AA wisdom, if I want to continue to experience this serenity, I have to "give it away" and share it with others. In a way, that's why

I'm writing this book. I want to share my holistic weight loss plan with you because it has worked so well for me and countless others. I want to hang onto my serenity and help you embark on your own journey to wellness.

5

Cleansing the Body

Steve came to see me because his high school football coach wanted him to lose some weight. Just 15-years-old, Steve weighed 305 pounds. He was grossly obese. His football coach wanted him to be big, but not that big. Steve was having trouble catching his breath at practice, and his coach wanted to see him lose some weight and get in shape.

I had Steve do a seven-day cleanse. A cleanse is a type of fast. Some people recommend strict water-only fasts, but the cleanse that I recommend supplies all the nutrients you need. Thus, I usually call it a cleanse rather than a fast because it's purpose is to cleanse your body (not to make you go hungry and suffer).

Nonetheless, Steve had a tough time that week. He experienced withdrawal symptoms as well as symptoms of toxicity. Typically, the more weight someone has to lose, the more toxic they are. During a cleanse, when those toxins are released by fat cells, they move into the bloodstream and poison the body. Steve suffered from headaches and fatigue all week.

But Steve made it through the cleanse, and at the end

of the week, he had lost a whopping 21 pounds! The next week, he had more energy than ever, and his performance on the field was better than ever. He continued to see me for weight management, kept working hard, and eventually got a football scholarship to a major college.

While not everyone agrees on cleansing methodology, virtually all health experts agree that cleansing is beneficial for the body. Cleansing allows the body to eliminate unwanted toxins and begin to heal.

Imagine if the air filters in your house were never changed, or if you never replaced the oil filter in your car. Eventually, this would lead to premature mechanical failure. The human body has its own filters. The main organs that filter toxins out of your body are the liver, kidneys, and intestines. A healthy cleanse will clean and repair these organs. If you're experiencing multiple symptoms of toxicity - fatigue, brain fog, headaches, inability to lose weight - then your body is telling you that it's time for a cleanse. Your symptoms are akin to your body's "check engine" light.

When toxins overcome your body, they are stored in fat cells and nerve tissue, like the brain. The more toxic the body, the more obese it becomes. If the body's filters are not given time to cleanse and regenerate, more fat is needed to handle these toxins. Eventually, this causes disease and catastrophic premature failure. Flushing toxins from your fat tissue will enable you to lose inches of fat during the cleanse process. Weight loss is a pleasant side effect of cleaning the body.

Fasting may be the world's oldest natural healing modality. It triggers healing on the cellular level. During the first couple of days of a cleanse, enzymes that are normally busy in the stomach become free to patrol the intestines and bloodstream, where they clean up waste matter like dead cells, unfriendly microbes, and pollutants. Your digestive organs get a much-needed rest, allowing their tissues to heal and rejuvenate. Your entire digestive tract will be thoroughly cleaned and rebalanced, and this will strengthen your immune system. After all, the majority of your immune systems is located within your gut. A cleanse allows your immune system to reboot and rebuild itself.

When I realized that I was addicted to food and need to detox my body to break my addiction, I tried the 21-day water fast that my daughter had completed. I didn't last the full 21 days. My energy levels plummeted, and I could feel the effects of toxins being released into my bloodstream. I quickly realized that a pure water fast would not work for most people.

Whenever people undertake a strict water cleanse, they run the risk of experiencing a Herxheimer reaction. When a lot of toxins are released, they kill off bacteria living in the gut, and these dying bacteria release toxins as well. A Herxheimer reaction can cause fever, chills, headaches, muscle aches and pains, and even skin lesions. A Herxheimer reaction also promotes inflammation. This type of "health crisis" just doesn't sound very healthy to me.

I knew I had to develop a healthy way to cleanse the body. My life depended on it. I started studying all different types of fasts and cleanses -- from juice fasts to herbal cleanses. During this process I contacted my close friend and colleague, Dr. Jeffrey Cartwright, a fellow chiropractor in Colorado. Dr. Cartwright was also looking for a healthy way to eliminate toxins from the body.

"My parents both died of cancer at a young age," Dr. Cartwright told me. "My mother struggled with breast cancer and my father had non-Hodgkins' lymphoma."

With a family history of cancer, Dr. Cartwright wanted to help people rid their bodies of the environmental toxins that cause disease. We had different reasons for beginning our separate quests, but we were looking for the same solution. We decided to work together to find that solution.

I like the way Dr. Cartwright thinks. He's an avid naturalist, and he reminds us that human beings are no different than other animals in a natural ecosystem. We're all part of the polluted environment.

"If we went fishing at a lake near your home and caught a fish with a big cancerous tumor, what would you think?" Dr. Cartwright asked me. "Would you say that we need to put toxic drugs into the water to prevent more tumors? Would you say that the fish needs surgery to remove necessary body parts? No! Most people would ask, 'What is the toxic environment of this lake and how can we clean it up to prevent future illness?' Why are we not asking the same question with regard to our own bodies?"

Dr. Cartwright and I began to study natural herbs and plant substances that can help the body eliminate toxins. After several years of research and experimentation, we developed a gentle yet highly effective cleansing and weight loss system.

This systems combines Ultra Cleanse, a nutrient formula that helps the body release the stored toxins that are preventing you from losing weight; Meta Boost, a natural metabolism booster to improve fat burning ability; and Energizer Protein Meal, a protein meal replacement to maintain energy levels and reduce fatigue during the cleanse.

The natural ingredients in the Ultra Cleanse formula attach to toxins and pull them from the tissue so that they can be flushed out of the body. This seven-day cleanse will flush out toxins and associated inflammation and restore balance to your body's internal environment.

The Ultra Cleanse formula is compounded with all the minerals and herbs you need to avoid a Herxheimer reaction. The Energizer Protein Meal also helps you to avoid the side effects associated with other detox programs.

"Most toxins are stored in your fat and brain tissue," Dr. Cartwright adds, "We designed a formula to help you think and feel better. The body uses fats to buffer the harmful effects of toxins. If you are toxic, you will maintain body fat. With our system, we can rid the toxins in the blood and fat cells and cleanse the liver and kidneys to improve their function of flushing toxins from the body. The result is improved health and a leaner body. The response has been tremendous! Most patients experience phenomenal weight loss."

The best thing about this cleanse, in practical terms, is that it can be done without sacrificing valuable time and energy. You don't have to take time off work or change your schedule.

Let me make it clear that our system is not a colon cleanse. (I never recommend products or procedures that I haven't tried myself, and that's why I don't recommend colon cleanses.) You will eliminate harmful toxins through your normal urine and bowel movements.

Since I started offering our cleanse to my patients, they've had tremendous success with weight loss. In fact, the success rate is around 70 percent for patients in my MET Right program. (Again, "MET Right" stands for Move Right, Eat Right, Think Right). I haven't come across another weight loss program with such a high success rate.

The average woman in my office loses 8 to 10 pounds during a seven-day cleanse, and the average man loses 10 to 12 pounds. I lost 13 pounds during my first cleanse, and my wife, who is a fairly small person, lost 17 pounds.

You're probably wondering what's inside the Ultra Cleanse formula and why it works so well. Unfortunately, I cannot tell you because the formula is proprietary. It's a trade secret.

Just kidding! The ingredients in the Ultra Cleanse formula are all natural, and there's no reason to keep them a secret. We want you to understand how it works. Here are the ingredients in the Ultra Cleanse:

Aloe Vera is a mixture of antibiotic, astringent, and coagulating agents, as well as vitamin C and vitamin B2. Aloe vera is a natural laxative that relieves bowel irritation and constipation. Preliminary studies show that aloe vera may improve glucose levels in diabetics and lower the chances of heart disease in patients with high cholesterol.

Alpha Lipolic Acid (ALA) is vitally important for

strengthening immunity and preventing many degenerative conditions such as heart disease. ALA is a powerful antioxidant that the body makes naturally. Antioxidants are substances that work by attacking free radicals (waste products created when the body turns food into energy.) Environmental toxins like ultraviolet rays, radiation, and toxic chemicals in cigarette smoke, car exhaust, and pesticides also generate free radicals. These free radicals cause harmful chemical reactions that can damage cells in the body, making it harder for the body to fight off infections and accelerating the aging process. Supplementing your natural supply of ALA will help the body eliminating free radicals and prevent cellular damage.

Amino Acid Blend (L-Carnitine, Glutamate, L-Methionine): Amino acids and proteins regulate nearly every biochemical reaction in the body. Amino acids are the building blocks used to form the proteins that make up muscles, bones, skin, hair, internal organs, and bodily fluids. Proteins regulate cell generation and repair, form antibodies to combat invading bacteria and viruses, assist the body's immune system, and assist in regulation of neurotransmitters and the transmission of chemical impulses in the central nervous system.

Calcium is essential for the proper development of bones and teeth as well as normal muscle activity (including heart function). Calcium aids the clotting process of the blood, stimulates enzymes in the digestive process, speeds the healing process, controls the conduction mechanism in the nerve tissues and is essential for proper utilization of phosphorus and vitamins A, C, and D.

According to the National Institutes of Health, many Americans consume less than half the amount of calcium recommended to build and maintain healthy bones. Heavy use of caffeine can diminish calcium levels; therefore, higher amounts of calcium may be needed if you drink a lot of coffee. Also, a diet high in protein can increase loss of calcium through the urine. Excessive intake of sodium, phosphates (from carbonated beverages) and alcohol, as well as the use of aluminum-containing antacids, also contribute to increased excretion of calcium.

Symptoms of calcium deficiency include muscle spasm or cramping, typically in hands or feet; hair loss (alopecia); dry skin and nails which may also become misshapen; numbness, tingling, or burning sensation around the mouth and fingers; nausea and vomiting; headaches; yeast infections (candidiasis); anxiety; convulsions/seizures; and poor tooth and bone development.

Choline is an essential nutrient normally grouped with the B vitamin complex. Choline assists in the transportation of fats in the body and prevents accumulation of fat in the liver. It is necessary for normal functioning of the kidneys and livers.

Chromium is an essential mineral that plays an important role in the metabolism of carbohydrates and fats. It works with insulin in the metabolism of sugar and increases the effectiveness of insulin by facilitating the transport of glucose into the cells. Chromium also transports protein where it is needed and aids in growth. It has been found to be beneficial in the prevention and treatment of high blood pressure. Chromium may help prevent diabetes, and it helps control total cholesterol and triglyceride levels. Chromium has demonstrated the ability to lower total and LDL ("bad") cholesterol levels and raise HDL ("good") cholesterol levels in the blood, particularly in people with high cholesterol. Chromium promotes weight loss, builds muscle, and reduces body fat.

Herbal Blend: Siberian ginseng has anti-stress effects, decreases fatigue, decreases the risk of atherosclerosis, and enhances mental and physical performance. American Ginseng enhances physical and mental performance and increases energy as well as resistance to harmful effects of stress and aging. Ginseng appears to reduce blood sugar levels and increases levels of high-density lipoprotein (HDL) cholesterol. Pau d'Arco is useful against cancer, diabetes, rheumatism, and ulcers. Fennel found to stimulate appetite, aid in digestion, beneficial for prevention of kidney stones, menopausal problems, nausea and obesity. Burdock Root purifies the blood, acts as a diuretic, and restores the liver. Peppermint relieves constipation, indigestion and cramps. Licorice is beneficial for relieving allergies, PMS, and menopausal problems. Guar Ana and Kola Nut are high in caffeine used to enhance thermogenesis (heat production and fat burning). Gymnema Sylverstre is an Ayurvedic treatment for diabetes. Cayenne is useful in treatment of skin afflictions, colds, pleurisy and kidney problems. Garcinia Cambogia suppresses the appetite and inhibits an enzyme involved in converting carbohydrates to fat. Cascara Sagrada is used in treatment of chronic constipation. Slippery Elm Bark is useful in treatment of afflictions affecting the bowels, kidney, bladder, stomach and lungs. Yucca used in the treatment for rheumatism and arthritis. Senna is known for its strong laxative effect.

Inositol is essential for the transportation of fat. It plays an important role in providing nourishment to the brain cells. Inositol also helps to lower cholesterol, promotes the growth of healthy hair, and helps prevent eczema. It has also been used to treat depression.

Niacin, or Vitamin B3, is important for proper blood circulation and healthy functioning of the nervous system. It maintains the normal functions of the gastrointestinal tract and is essential for the proper metabolism of proteins and carbohydrates. Niacian also helps to maintain healthy skin and dilation of blood capillaries. It is essential for synthesis of the sex hormones estrogen, progesterone, and testosterone, as well as the synthesis of cortisone, thyroxin, and insulin. Niacin also assists in maintaining mental and emotional well-being.

Pantothenic Acid, or Vitamin B5, is necessary for the

metabolism of all macronutrients (proteins, carbs, and fats).

Riboflavin, or Vitamin B2, is essential for the metabolism of carbohydrates. It helps keep mucous membranes healthy, and it's essential for growth and general health. Riboflavin functions as a part of a group of enzymes that are involved in the metabolism of carbohydrates, fats, and proteins. It's involved in a number of chemical reactions and is essential for normal tissue maintenance. Riboflavin aids digestion and helps in the functioning of the nervous system. It prevents constipation and promotes healthy skin, nails, and hair. Riboflavin strengthens the mucous lining of the mouth, lips, and tongue. It also plays an important role in eye health and in counteracting the tendency towards glaucoma. Vitamin B2 provides vigor and helps preserve the appearance and feeling of youth.

Royal Jelly is secreted by bees and fed to the larvae. It's called "royal" jelly because only a future queen bee receives a large amount of it. It contains the B vitamins as well as vitamins A, C, D, and E, together with amino acids, minerals, and antibacterial components. It's known to strengthen the immune system and treat conditions such as fatigue, low sex drive, liver disease, stomach ulcers, kidney disease, inflammation, and skin problems.

Sodium is involved in electrolyte balance and required for normal nerve and muscle function, so it's important to maintain healthy levels of sodium during a cleanse.

Thiamin, or Vitamin B1, is required for the metabolism of carbohydrates and normal nerve and heart function. It promotes growth, protects the heart muscle, and stimulates brain function. Thiamin plays an important role in the normal functioning of the entire nervous system, aids digestion, and has a mild diuretic effect. It improves peristalsis and prevents constipation, and it helps to maintain a normal red blood cell count and improves circulation.

Individuals with thiamine deficiency have difficulty digesting carbohydrates. As a result, a substance called pyruvic acid builds up in the bloodstream, causing a loss of mental alertness, difficulty breathing, and heart damage. In general, thiamine supplements are primarily used to treat this deficiency known as beriberi. Vitamin B1 reduces fatigue, increases stamina, and prevents premature aging and senility by increasing mental alertness.

Vitamin B6 is essential for the metabolism of amino acids and fatty acids, for normal nerve function, and for the formation of red blood cells. It helps keep skin healthy and activates many enzymes and enzyme systems. Vitamin B6 is involved in the production of antibodies, which protect against bacterial diseases, and helps in the healthy functioning of the nervous system and brain. It is essential for the normal reproductive process and healthy pregnancies. Vitamin B6 prevents nervous and skin disorders while providing protection against high cholesterol, certain types of heart disease and diabetes. It also regulates the balance between sodium and potassium in the body and is required for absorption of vitamin B12 and magnesium.

Vitamin B12 is essential for the production and regeneration of red blood cells. It is needed for the proper functioning of the central nervous system. It improves concentration, memory, balance, and helps to relieve irritability. It is also necessary for proper utilization of fats, carbohydrates and proteins. Vitamin B12 is involved in many vital metabolic and enzymatic processes, including the metabolism of folic acid. It is also necessary for immune cells to mature into active disease-fighters.

Vitamin C is essential for the formation of bone and connective tissue. It helps the body absorb iron and is an antioxidant that protects cells against damage by free radicals. Vitamin C is necessary for the maintenance of bones and proper functioning of the adrenal and thyroid glands. This vitamin promotes healing and protects against all forms of stress, both physical and mental. It provides protection against harmful effects of toxic chemicals in our environment, food, and water and counteracts the toxic effects of drugs.

For a full review of all the medical research related to the above ingredients, please see "Nutritional Research" at www.novolife.net.

Because of the potential for side effects and interactions with medications, dietary supplements should be taken only under the supervision of a knowledgeable healthcare provider.

If our world weren't so polluted, your body would be able to process natural toxins and prevent toxic overload. However, in our world, natural toxins combined with man-made toxins have created widespread toxic overload. Detoxification is necessary to cleanse your body and restore healthy function.

We developed our program as a unique cleanse system because it is easy to use, and you can maintain your normal, busy schedule without suffering from fatigue or a healing crisis. The Ultra Cleanse formula stimulates the release of toxins by enhancing your body's natural detox pathways, while the medical-food-grade meal replacement provides energy in the form of a delicious protein shake with a low glycemic index. (Okay, so the shake is not exactly delicious, but it's not bad.) This will give you the nutritional support you need throughout the cleanse, while the Meta Boost capsules will naturally boost your body's fat metabolism.

Water: Flusher of Toxins

Dr. Cartwright and I have put together the best cleanse system available using the most helpful nutritional supplements in the world - but these supplements pale in comparison to the power of pure water. Water is the true healer.

Dr. Fereydoon Batmanghelidj, MD, author of The Body's Many Cries for Water, writes: "Every function inside the body is regulated by and depends on water. Water must be available to carry vital elements, oxygen, hormones, and chemical messengers to all parts of the body. Without sufficient water to wet all parts equally, some more remote parts of the body will not receive the vital elements that water supplies. Water is also needed to carry toxic waste away from the cells. In fact, there are at least 50 reasons why the body needs sufficient water on a regular, everyday basis."

In the past, only a couple hundred years ago, water was the only thing you needed for a fast. Today, however, our toxic world has overloaded our filtration systems, and our bodies need more help in the cleansing process. Using proper nutritional support can assist your body in this process and provide a new beginning.

When you start your cleanse, be sure to drink at least six tall glasses of purified water a day, in addition to your protein shakes. The water, when combined with nutrients, will cleanse your system and flush away toxins.

When your cleanse begins to take effect, your body will become more alkaline; this will boost the efficiency of enzymatic reactions and allow your liver to release waste products faster. Your body will finally be able to let go of excess waste and excess fat. You'll be amazed at the results.

Flushing Out Toxic Medications

This week I have 14 patients coming into my clinic to start a cleanse. Whenever patients begin a cleanse, I always go over their current medications and supplements to check for possible interactions and side effects. I also tell them that they need to tell their medical doctor they are beginning the cleanse.

So many people in our society have become accustomed to treating all of their symptoms with a pill. Many of my patients are amazed to discover that they don't need as much medication after their cleanse. A cleanse strengthens the immune system and allows the body to heal itself.

In virtually all cases, patients who are taking prescription medication will be overmedicated during or after a cleanse. That's why it is imperative that they talk to their medical doctor. Many diabetes medications, for example, lower blood sugar. But a patient's blood sugar will go down naturally during a cleanse. The continued use of medications could cause the blood sugar to drop too low. Always talk to your doctor before starting a cleanse. You may be able to cut your medications in half. Also, if you're cleansing your body to eliminate toxic chemicals, you don't want to keep dumping toxic chemicals into your body throughout the cleanse; that's counterproductive. Talk to your medical doctor and see if you can reduce or pause your medications during the cleanse. You may find that you never have to resume taking them!

A cleanse may lower your blood pressure, your cholesterol, your triglycerides, and your blood sugar. You may find that your energy levels drop initially, but a cleanse will ultimately increase your energy levels.

"Fasting also brings about an energy boost," writes Dr. Don Colbert, MD, author of Toxic Relief. "Most people eating the typical American diet have a toxic buildup within their cells. This results in the mitochondria (the energy factory inside each cell) being unable to effectively produce energy for the body. Over time fatigue, irritability, and lethargy set in. But when we fast, cellular waste is removed and cells can begin making energy again."

A cleanse will also break your addiction to fast food (at least temporarily). For me, that was the most powerful and life-changing benefit. I no longer craved burgers and fries! My body had been addicted to refined sugar and fat, and the cleanse broke that addiction. I could actually enjoy steamed broccoli, whereas before, whenever I ate steamed broccoli, I was also fantasizing about a side of fries.

Whenever I feel myself slipping - for instance, if I have a burger or slice of pizza over the weekend and find myself craving fast food - then I do a mini-cleanse to nip the addiction in the bud. This is the most effective weight loss system I've tried - and I've tried them all!

Flushing Out Toxic Organisms & Biological Waste

Fasting or cleansing will also alter your intestinal microflora, or the balance of the microorganisms living inside your gut. Candida, for example, the yeast-like fungal organisms in the gut, can become toxic in large numbers. Candida produce toxins like acetaldehyde, a waste product that can effect neurological, immune, and endocrine systems.

Cleansing will balance out the population of candida in your gut by starving them to death. Candida (and many other potentially harmful organisms) live off sugar. Once you cut out your sugar intake, the organisms will begin to die off, and your immune system can eliminate them.

An intestinal tract that's clogged with toxic sludge is a prime breeding ground for harmful bacteria and parasites like intestinal worms. By priming the immune system, cleansing will help your body eliminate these opportunistic organisms. I recommend two seven-day cleanses per year for everyone. I normally do one cleanse during the spring and one during the fall with several mini-cleanses in between.

"The main benefit of fasting is that it gives your digestive system a chance to rest," writes Dr. Colbert, author of Toxic Relief. "Our body uses a lot of energy every day in digesting, absorbing and assimilating food. When we fast, our digestive tract is given a chance to rest and repair. This in turn gives our liver, the body's largest and most effective filter, an opportunity to catch up on its job of removing toxins.

"The body's primary channels of elimination include the kidneys and urinary tract, the colon, the lungs and the skin. These are the avenues through which our body gets rid of toxins. Think about it. Our body has sixty to one hundred trillion cells, and each one takes in nutrients and produces waste. Fasting allows each cell to dump its waste and be able to function at peak capacity. This enables cells to heal, repair, and be strengthened. Additionally, fatty tissues release chemicals and toxins during fasting that are then broken down by the liver, excreted by the kidneys and through the bowel.

"Periodic, short-term fasting will also strengthen your immune system and help you live longer. As your body detoxifies, your skin will eventually become clearer, the whites of your eyes usually become whiter, and your mental functioning usually improves."

Auxiliary Avenues of Detox

The lymphatic system is similar to the cardiovascular system. The cardiovascular system circulates blood, and the lymphatic system circulates lymph. While blood vessels carry nutrients to the tissues, lymphatic vessels absorb excess fluid from the blood as well as waste products, bacteria, cellular debris, and toxins. Lymph nodes filter out toxins and germs. When your lymph nodes are swollen, it's a sign that your white blood cells are hard at work.

Unlike the heart-driven cardiovascular system, the lymphatic system does not have a central pump. Lymph flow relies on muscle movement. Therefore, a sedentary lifestyle can lead to an accumulation of toxins in the lymph.

You can help your body detox during a cleanse by making sure that your lymph is flowing. Regular exercise is the best way to stimulate lymph flow. Lymphatic drainage is a special type of massage therapy in which the therapist manually initiates the flow of lymph. Most types of massage therapy will help to stimulate lymph flow.

Baths and showers can be effective methods of detoxing, too. Take long, hot baths, and pour sea salt and baking soda into the bath to enhance the detox process. Use a cup of baking soda and one to two cups of sea salt or epsom salts. Soak for at least 20 minutes. Breathe deeply and relax.

Contrast showers will also help stimulate the flow of blood and lymph. A contrast shower is nothing more than a shower in which you alternate between hot and cold water. Start with hot water, blast yourself with cold water for about a minute, go back to hot, do one more cold blast, and finish with hot water. You can also give yourself a lymphatic drainage massage of sorts when washing and drying. Vigorously scrub and towel-dry every inch of your body. Get that lymph moving; it's not going anywhere on its own.

Finally, sweating is a great way to eliminate toxins. Native Americans used sweat lodges to open their skin pores, allowing toxins to stream out. Today, you may have a hard time finding a sweat lodge, but your local gym probably has a sauna room. Of course, regular exercise will make you sweat, too. Exercise doesn't have to be painful and boring. Find a fun activity that makes you sweat, and do it often.

Spiritual Cleansing

Fasting, or cleansing, will detoxify your body, melt away fat, and improve your health and wellbeing. Many people also fast for spiritual reasons. In the Book of Matthew, Jesus says that Christians should give alms, pray, and fast. I attend services at a Methodist Church, and my church has taught us how to give and pray, but I never heard anything about fasting. So I asked my minister about it - and the next thing I knew, I was standing before the whole congregation, giving a lecture on spiritual cleansing.

I found 32 references to fasting in the Bible (and I'm sure I missed a few). In the Biblical sense, fasting is a form of self-sacrifice that makes one humble and more open to God's will. Moses fasted for 40 days before her received the 10 commandments; Daniel fasted for 21 days before he received his vision; Elijah fasted for 40 days before he spoke with God; and Jesus fasted for 40 days before he began his ministry.

Now, you probably won't get any spiritual benefits from fasting if that's not what you're seeking. Cleansing for spiritual reasons must go hand in hand with prayer or meditation. Fasting can in fact supercharge prayer and facilitate a closer relationship with God. I've found that my religious patients who fast for spiritual reasons as well as health reasons will often have more success with weight loss. Whenever they are tempted to eat junk food, they can turn to prayer as a source of inner strength. This helps some people get past the cravings.

Spiritual cleansing is not just a Christian tradition. Nearly all major religions practice some form of fasting. Muslims fast during Ramadan. Jews fast on Yom Kippur. Hindus fasts several times throughout the year. All the main branches of Buddhism practice fasting as a means of freeing the mind.

In The Power of Prayer and Fasting, author Marilyn Hickey writes, "What I have seen repeatedly through the years -- not only in the Scriptures but in countless personal stories that others have told me -- is that periods of fasting and prayer produce great spiritual results, many of which fall into the realm of a breakthrough. What wasn't a reality . . . suddenly was. What hadn't worked . . . suddenly did. The unwanted situation or object that was there . . . suddenly wasn't there. The relationship that was unloving . . . suddenly was loving. The job that hadn't materialized . . . suddenly did."

Whether you or a religious person or not, cleansing can clear your mind and lift your spirits. Once you flush the toxins out of your nervous system and brain tissue, you'll begin to feel and think differently. You may find that cleansing seems to shine a light on hidden gems in your life that you didn't notice before. A major Japanese study found that a 10-day cleanse improved or cured depression in 90 percent of patients.

I'm a neophyte when it comes to the benefits of spiritual fasting. When I spoke at my church, I really didn't know what I was talking about. I just rattled off what I knew about cleansing for health reasons and tried to apply that knowledge to spiritual cleansing. I wasn't sure if I was making any sense or getting through to people. But some time later, people began to approach me to tell me that they had tried spiritual cleansing and that miracles had occurred because of it. And now I'm scheduled to speak at several churches! I'm still learning about spiritual cleansing; I don't know everything about it, but I do know that it can be a powerful form of worship, especially when combined with prayer.

Breaking the Fast

After your cleanse ends, don't go out for pizza or burgers! At the end of a fast, your stomach will be low on digestive secretions and enzymes. A greasy meal would clog up your system immediately and could cause violent reactions like extreme vomiting. After your fast, avoid any foods that are difficult to digest - processed food, meat, and dairy. Even a piece of toast can land in the newly refurbished digestive system with the weight of a brick.

I recommend that patients end their cleanse with small servings of raw, organic fruit and vegetables. Fresh fruit and vegetables still have their natural enzymes intact; these enzymes will assist in the digestion process. Cooking destroys these enzymes, so it's best to stick with raw food immediately following a fast, although a bit of vegetable soup won't hurt if you're in the mood for some hot food. Eat very lightly for a few days, and slowly increase your daily intake of food. This will allow your digestive secretions to build back up to normal levels. Continue to drink plenty of water after the cleanse.

You may find that your sense of taste has improved after the fast, but you must resist the urge to overeat. You don't want to reverse all the health benefits as soon as your fast ends! Enjoy your new feeling of lightness and try to make it last.

You have broken your addiction to junk food. Congratulations! Now take advantage of your enhanced sense of taste by exploring the subtle flavors of various fresh fruits and vegetables.

6

Eat Right

Betty came to see me because of her back pain. During her first visit I asked, "What kind of medications are you taking?"

"Well, I can't tell you off the top of my head," she said.

"Okay," I said. "Just bring in your medications next week. We'll look at all of them, and I'll enter them into my database."

The next week, Betty came in with a brown paper grocery bag full of pill bottles. This was one of the large grocery bags, mind you, not one of the small ones. We dumped the bottles out on my desk and started going over them one by one.

"I take three of these in the morning," Betty said, holding up a bottle then dropping it on the opposite side of the desk. "I take this twice a day. I take one of these a day. I take this one every other day. I think I'm supposed to take this one once every other day, too, but sometimes I forget. And this one - well, I'm not really sure what this one is for."

I was sitting there with my notepad, furiously scribbling away, trying to keep up with Betty's litany of medications.

By the time we finished, I had compiled a list adding up

to 72 pills a day! Not all of these were prescription drugs - some were vitamins and supplements - but the vast majority had been prescribed by one of Betty's three medical doctors.

"This has got to be malpractice," I thought. *Talk about toxic overload!*

I'll admit, Betty had a lot of health problems. She was pushing 70; she'd had a recent back surgery; she had diabetes and heart disease, and she was overweight. She had her fair share of problems. But nobody should be taking 72 pills a day. That's just asking for trouble.

Betty was a punctual patient. She had never missed an appointment, so when she didn't show up one day, I asked my assistant to give her a call.

"She's in the hospital," my assistant told me. I picked up the phone to talk to her son.

"What happened?" I asked.

Her son told me that Betty had taken her cat's medication by mistake, and she was in the hospital getting her stomach pumped! (I can't see how the cat's medication could hurt her any more than the rest of the pills she was taking.)

This is how crazy our world has become.

The typical medical doctor has only two solutions to offer a sick patient: prescription drugs or surgery. More often than not, patients receive a prescription for a toxic drug that will only contribute to the body's toxic load. Prescription drugs might treat the symptom, but there's a good chance that they'll create even more symptoms through side effects. Moreover, medications treat symptoms without treating the underlying cause of illness.

Hippocrates, the father of modern medicine, had it right: Let food be your medicine.

Unfortunately, in my clinic, the average patient over 60 is on at least six different prescription medications. They're suffering from toxic overload not only because of the toxins in their environment and their food but also because of the drugs they're taking.

What is the underlying cause of illness? For most people,

it's a sedentary lifestyle combined with a poor diet and toxic overload. My weight loss program "MET Right" teaches people to move right, eat right, and think right. In this chapter, you'll learn how to eat your way to wellness.

Your seven-day cleanse will temporarily break your addiction to refined foods that are high in flavor, fat, and carbs but low in nutrition. This will allow you to start a new, healthy diet consisting of unrefined, whole foods. If you want to lose weight, you need to eat foods that have high nutrient densities, foods that will promote an alkaline rather than acidic pH level in your body, and foods that will deflame rather than inflame your body.

Nutrient Dense Foods

Most Americans get the majority of their calories from processed foods - soda, genetically engineered milk, margarine, white bread made with high-fructose corn syrup, corn-fed beef and chicken, and refined sugars. These foods are not natural. They are high in calories and low in nutrition, giving them low nutrient densities. They are the primary cause of the obesity epidemic, and they're killing us! A study in the *New England Journal of Medicine* reported that more than 85 percent of Americans between the ages of 21 and 39 already have signs of atherosclerosis in their coronary arteries.

If you want to lose weight, you have to cut out refined foods, including bread, bagels, and pasta. Chicken and pasta is not a healthy meal, especially if you want to lose weight.

In *Eat to Live*, Dr. Fuhrman, MD, explains, "The combination of fat and refined carbohydrates has an extremely powerful effect on driving the signals that promote fat accumulation on the body. Refined foods cause a swift and excessive rise in blood sugar, which in turn triggers insulin surges to drive the sugar out of the blood and into our cells. Unfortunately, insulin also promotes the storage of fat on the body and encourages your fat cells to swell."

"Eating refined carbohydrates - as opposed to complex carbohydrates in their natural state - causes the body's 'set point' for body weight to increase. Your 'set point' is the weight the body tries to maintain through the brain's control of hormonal messengers. When you eat refined fats (oils) or refined carbohydrates such as white flour and sugar, the fat-storing hormones are produced in excess, raising the set point. To further compound the problem, because so much of the vitamin and mineral content of these foods has been lost during processing, you naturally crave more food to make up for the missing nutrients."

I recommend that all of my patients buy a copy of *Eat to Live* and read it thoroughly. Dr. Fuhrman outlines exactly which foods you need to eat and which foods you need to avoid if you want to lose weight. In a nutshell, you should eat foods with high nutrient densities and avoid those with low nutrient densities.

Raw, leafy green vegetables (like romaine lettuce, kale, collards, spinach, and chard) have the highest nutrient densities. You should try to eat one pound of raw greens and one pound of cooked greens a day. If you fill up on nutrient-dense greens, you won't crave junk food, and your body will be getting all the nutrients it needs.

On the nutrient density scale, leafy greens are followed by solid green vegetables (like artichokes, asparagus, broccoli, cabbage, cucumber, peas, green peppers, zucchini), which may be eaten raw or steamed. Non-green, non-starchy vegetables include eggplant, mushrooms, onions, tomatoes, red and yellow peppers, cauliflower. These vegetables, along with beans and fresh fruits, can be eaten freely.

Try to eat two large salads every day, and add vegetables, beans, and fruit to your salad. Eat until you are satisfied. Do not allow yourself to get hungry!

Starchy vegetables (potatoes, squash, pumpkin, corn, carrots), whole grains (barley, buckwheat, oats, brown rice, wild rice, quinoa), and raw nuts and seeds should be eaten in moderation because their nutrient densities are lower, and they are higher in calories. Nuts offer health benefits, but you shouldn't eat more than a handful a day. Limit starchy vegetables and whole grains to no more than a cup a day.

Let's look at some of Dr. Fuhrman's recommendations in more detail. The following 10 foods have high nutrient density scores (on a scale of 1 to 1000), and you can eat as much of them as you want:

Kale: 1000 - Kale tops the list of nutrient dense foods. Before I read Eat to Live, I don't think I had ever eaten kale. Now I eat it several times a week. It's actually a type of cabbage, and it's full of vitamins and anti-inflammatory phytonutrients. Kale is hearty enough to store in the freezer, so you can always stay stocked up. Some people think it actually tastes sweeter after it's frozen. You can steam or boil kale. Boil it gently for just a few minutes until the leaves turn bright green. I normally eat it with fresh garlic and lemon juice drizzled on top.

Collards: 916 - Collard greens are popular in the South, where they're normally cooked with butter or another form of fat like smoked and salted meats. ("Fatback" never sounded very appetizing to me.) Fortunately, you can prepare collards without the extra fat. While Southern chefs generally boil collards for a long time, I gently boil it until the leaves turn bright green - just about five minutes or so.

Spinach: 886 - As Popeye's favorite health food, spinach gave him big muscles while protecting him against osteoporosis, heart disease, colon cancer, arthritis, and other diseases. You can eat spinach raw, steamed, or boiled. My salads usually contain a mixture of spinach and lettuce.

Bok Choy: 839 - Oh boy! Bok choy, also known as Chinese cabbage, is becoming more popular because of its nutritional value. A cup of bok choy contains only 20 calories; it's also a good source of calcium as well as vitamins C and A. Both the leaves and stems are edible.

You'll want to chop them into pieces before cooking. Steam bok choy or gently boil it for a few minutes.

Romaine Lettuce: 462 - Romaine is my favorite type of lettuce. It's too bad that this heart-healthy leaf is normally served with croutons, cheese, and high-fat dressing! For a healthier salad, leave off the croutons and cheese and order a low-fat dressing on the side. Or skip the dressing altogether and add flavor to your salad with vegetables and fruits. Fresh-squeezed citrus juice makes a delicious salad dressing.

Bell Peppers: 420 - Sweet bell peppers provide colorful protection against free radicals that promote aging. As the mature, ripened versions of green peppers, red and yellow peppers contain more vitamin C, lycopene, and carotene than green peppers. But you don't have to avoid green peppers! With a more tart flavor, green peppers still have a nutrient density score of 295 (and they're usually cheaper at the grocery store).

Boston Lettuce: 412 - Boston lettuce, also known as butter lettuce, is very tender with a subtle flavor. It's packed with vitamins and minerals as well as lactucarium, a chemical with opium-like properties that can help treat insomnia and spasms. Next time you're having trouble sleeping, eat a big Boston lettuce salad for dinner.

Broccoli: 395 - Men who eat broccoli more than once a week are 45% less likely to develop aggressive prostate cancer. Good enough for me. Pass the broccoli, please! Cruciferous vegetables like broccoli and cauliflower offer significant protection against cancer. Sprinkle lemon juice and sesame seeds over lightly steamed broccoli for a healthy, tasty side dish, or add broccoli florets to your salad.

Artichokes: 334 - Artichokes are virtually fat-free and high in folic acid, vitamin C, and magnesium. If you've never cooked artichokes before, you might be a little confused when you get home from the grocery store. To prepare an artichoke, first cut off the thorny tips of the leaves. You can cut off the stem or leave it attached. (The stem is a little bitter, but some people enjoy it.) Rinse the artichokes, and then steam for about 30 minutes until the outer leaves can be easily pulled off. Pull off the petals one at a time, and use your teeth to remove the soft portion of the petal; discard the rest. Once you've eaten all the petals, use a spoon to remove the artichoke heart. This is my favorite part.

Cabbage: 329 - Cabbage provides protection against cancer, Alzheimer's disease, and heart disease. Slice or chop the cabbage to release myrosinase enzymes that activate cancer-fighting phytonutrients. Cooking the cabbage will denature theses enzymes, so eat your cabbage raw or lightly steamed to get the most nutritional value out of it.

All leaf lettuces, chard, parsley, and daikon also have high nutrient density scores. Eat as many leafy greens as possible! Every additional bite will supply you with more health-promoting nutrients.

Many fruits have high nutrient density scores as well, like strawberries (254), cherries (197), blueberries (155), and oranges (130). Some high-calorie fruits, on the other hand, have lower scores. Bananas, for instance, have a nutrient density score of only 36.

Opt for whole fruits over fruit juice whenever possible. The whole fruit contains more nutrients and fiber. Apple juice, for example, has a score of 30, but apples have a score of 91.

Most whole grains, beans, and starchy vegetables have scores between 50 and 100, and you should eat them in moderation.

Olive oil, often touted as a health food, actually has a very low nutrient density score. After all, it's 100 percent refined fat! If you want to lose weight, you should avoid all refined oils. Following are 10 foods with low nutrient densities which you should avoid:

Soft drinks: 0.6 - Soda has a nutrient density score of less than one, but I think it should actually be in the negative! Soft drinks, even diet soft drinks, should be considered health hazards.

"The United States ranks first among countries in soft drink consumption," according to the *Encyclopedia of Natural Medicine.* "The per-capita consumption of soft drinks is in excess of 150 quarts per year, or about three quarts per week.

"Soft drinks have long been suspected of leading to lower calcium levels and higher phosphate levels in the blood. When phosphate levels are high and calcium levels are low, calcium is pulled out of the bones. The phosphate content of soft drinks like Coca-Cola and Pepsi is very high, and they contain virtually no calcium.

"Soft drink consumption in children poses a significant risk factor for impaired calcification of growing bones."

If you want to gain weight and increase your risk of developing osteoporosis, keep drinking cola; otherwise, skip the soda or replace it with water. If you're addicted to the caffeine, substitute green tea for soda.

Olive Oil: 2 - Compared to animal fats like butter and hydrogenated vegetable oils, monosaturated olive oil is certainly the healthier choice. However, as refined fat, olive oil has a very low nutrient density. If you're trying to lose weight, you should avoid consumption of refined fats. The Mediterranean diet promotes the use of olive oil, but the health benefits of this diet stem from a high consumption of fruits and vegetables rather than a high consumption of olive oil.

Ice Cream: 6 - Most ice cream is high in fat, sugar, and salt. Sure, it tastes great, but it can be highly addictive, and it has a low nutrient density. Ice cream should be a rare treat eaten in small quantities.

Potato Chips: 13 - Potato chips are high in cancer-causing acrylamide, fat, salt, and calories. Like ice cream, potato chips can be highly addictive, and they don't provide proper nutrition.

Ground Beef: 17 - The average American eats 67 pounds of ground beef a year. A high intake of ground beef increases the risk of cancer as well as heart disease. A recent National Cancer Institute study found a 30 percent increase in the risk of fatality directly correlating with the consumption of red meat and processed meat. It's okay to eat ground beef in moderation every once in a while. I try to limit my consumption of red meat to no more than once every couple of weeks, and I try to select free-range, grass-fed beef. With a nutrient density score of 46, shrimp is a much healthier choice for meat.

Cheese: 18 - According to the Center for Science in the Public Interest (CSPI), cheese consumption has nearly tripled since 1970, making it the nation's number one source of saturated fat. A high intake of saturated fat clogs arteries and leads to heart disease.

"Americans are eating far too much fatty cheese," said Margo Wootan of the CSPI. "Unfortunately, it's everywhere: on sandwiches, on lean chicken, on salads, and even on fries. And it's doing even more damage to our hearts than beef or butter."

Peanut Butter: 21 - Believe it or not, there's a popular book called *The Peanut Butter Diet.* Maybe I should really write a book called *The Pizza Diet!* Peanut butter is high in fat, high in calories, and relatively low in nutrients. If you want to lose weight, peanut butter is not your friend. It should be eaten in moderation if at all. And if you do eat peanut butter, choose the organic variety.

White Bread: 21 - Have you noticed that these foods with low nutrient densities are the most popular foods in America (while many Americans have never even tried kale or bok choy)? White bread is high in carbs, has limited nutritional value, and has been stripped of its natural fiber. Oh, and most white bread contains high-fructose corn syrup! And guess what - whole wheat bread isn't much better for you; whole wheat bread has a nutrient density score of 25. Skip the bread if you want to lose weight. Replace sandwiches with salads.

White Pasta: 22 - Sorry, pasta lovers. The carbs in refined white flour spikes your blood sugar without offering much in the way of nutrition.

Whole Milk: 22 - Wait a minute . . . Doesn't milk do a body good? Not quite. Milk is high in fat and low in nutrients. Sure, milk provides calcium, but so do green vegetables (and milk promotes the loss of calcium in the urine). Most milk is also tainted with genetically engineered hormones and antibiotics. If you must drink milk, choose organic skim milk, which has a nutrient density score of 43.

Inflammation Information

Refined grains and dairy are the two most inflammatory foods out there. Dr. David Seaman, DC, author of deflame. com, writes that the following conditions (among others) are driven by diet-induced inflammation: aches and pain, osteoarthritis, rheumatoid arthritis, osteoporosis, acne, aging, syndrome X, diabetes, cancer, heart disease, peripheral vascular disease, stroke, Alzhemier's disease, Parkinson's disease, psoriasis, eczema, and multiple sclerosis.

I've had the privilege of attending a few lectures by Dr. Seaman, and I've got to tell you: at first, I didn't like what he had to say. My favorite food in the whole world is bread, you see. I argued with this man vehemently. *Say it aint so,* I pleaded. In the end, Dr. Seaman's research convinced me that bread and refined grains in general should not be consumed frequently.

Refined grains have high glycemic indexes that increase blood sugar and insulin levels. Over time, frequent consumption of refined grains can lead to diabetes, heart disease, and cancer. Whole grains, on the other hand, contain anti-inflammatory fiber. But even whole grains contain gluten, lectins, phytates, a high ration of omega-6 to omega-3 fats - and they promote an acidic pH level in the body - all of which contribute to inflammation.

"These several pro-inflammatory factors outweigh the

fiber benefits of whole grains, and we get significantly more fiber on a caloric basis from fruits and vegetables," writes Dr. Seaman. "Accordingly, we should try to avoid eating grains. If you would like a starchy food, potatoes are our best choice."

Next time you eat a meal, look at your plate and ask yourself: *Am I eating inflammation? Am I eating food that will cause pain and disease? Do I want to experience the pain that this food will cause me?*

As a combination of refined grains and dairy, macaroni and cheese is one of the worst foods you could eat. It's also one of the worst foods you could feed to a child, yet it's one of the most popular children's foods.

Inflammatory foods plus toxins creates poor health and a shortened lifespan. This is a bold statement to make, but if you deflame and eliminate toxins, you will probably never die of cancer, heart disease, or diabetes, nor will you suffer from the pain of fibromyalgia. You will live a long, healthy life. They say that fibromyalgia is incurable, but if you get rid of the inflammation that's causing it, then you won't have fibromyalgia any more. A cleanse will help you get rid of toxins and inflammation, and better health and increased longevity are the results.

According to Dr. Seaman's Deflaming Guidelines, the following foods are inflammatory and should be avoided:

• *All grains and grain products, including white bread, whole wheat bread, pasta, cereal, pretzels, crackers, and any other product made with grains or flours from grains, which includes most desserts and packaged snacks.*

• *Partially hydrogenated oils (trans fats) found in margarine, deep fried foods (French fries, etc.) and most all packaged foods.*

• *Corn oil, safflower oil, sunflower oil, cottonseed oil, peanut oil, soybean oil, and foods made with these oils such as mayonnaise, tartar sauce, margarine, salad dressings, and many packaged foods.*

• *Soda and sugar are inflammatory.*

• *If you eat dairy or soy, they should be consumed as condiments, not staples.*

• *Meat and eggs from grain-fed animals (domesticated animal products). Modern meat is problematic because the animals are obese and unhealthy; they are loaded with saturated fats and contain too many pro-inflammatory omega-6 fatty acids. Grass-fed meat or wild game are our best choices. Otherwise, we should eat lean meat, skinless chicken, turkey, omega-3 eggs and fish. Lean cuts of meat and lean hamburger meat are available at most grocery stores, and even extra-lean is sometimes available.*

If you eat a diet consisting primarily of unrefined plant foods with high nutrient densities, then you will naturally avoid the most inflammatory foods. Fruits, vegetables, raw nuts and seeds, and lean meats from grass-fed or wild animals are anti-inflammatory.

Acid-Base Balance

As your body temperature must remain right around 98.6 degrees Fahrenheit to maintain your health, your body's pH level must remain right around 7.35 (slightly alkaline). The body is very sensitive to changes in pH. When it becomes too acidic
(a condition known as acidosis), the body has several mechanisms for restoring acid-base balance.

In *The New Nutrition,* Michael Colgan explains that acidosis "destroys bones because the body has to steal alkalizing minerals from them to keep the blood pH from dropping into the acid range." A high-fat, high-sugar diet produces excess acids in the body, and such a diet can lead to osteoporosis over time.

The body also maintains its acid-base balance by storing excess acids in fat tissue. Dr. Robert Young, author of *The pH Miracle for Weight Loss,* writes: "The pH level (the acid-alkaline measurement) of our internal fluids affects every cell in our bodies. Extended acid imbalances of any kind are not well tolerated by the body. Indeed, the entire metabolic process depends on a balanced internal alkaline environment. A chronically over-acidic pH corrodes body tissue, slowly eating into the 60,000 miles of veins and arteries like acid eating into marble. If left unchecked, it will interrupt all cellular activities and functions, from the beating of your heart to the neural firing of your brain. In summary, over-acidification interferes with life itself, leading to all sickness and disease!"

Because acids can be so harmful, the body treats them like toxins. Fat tissue stores excess acids in the same way that it stores toxins. A diet that's high in acid-forming foods makes it difficult to lose weight. When you detox to eliminate excess acids and start to eat an alkalizing diet, weight loss will follow. Dr. Young explains, "If your food and drink are alkaline, all the acid-binding fat will just melt right off. There will be no need for the body to hold onto it anymore."

What are acid-forming foods? The primary acid-forming foods are meat, cheese, bread, butter, grains, sugar, soft drinks, and artificial sweeteners. Some healthy foods like certain beans and mushrooms form acids, too. There's nothing inherently wrong with an acid-forming food, but the typical American diet contains far too many acid-forming foods and not enough alkalizing foods.

Alkalizing foods include fruits and vegetables. Note that an acidic food does not necessarily form acids in the body. Citrus fruits, for example, are acidic foods, but they have an alkalizing affect on the body.

If you avoid processed food and eat a diet consisting primarily of unrefined plant foods, your body won't have a problem with its acid-base balance, and you'll be able to lose weight more easily. A plant-based diet will also provide anti-inflammatory foods with high nutrient densities.

Now that you know what to eat and what *not* to eat, let's discuss how to carry out your new diet plan. It won't be easy. You'll be tempted by junk food on every corner, and chances are, you've been eating an unhealthy diet for a long time. Here are some tips to help you incorporate your newfound knowledge about food into your diet:

Eat a big salad for lunch and dinner before you eat anything else. Raw leafy greens should make up the bulk of your salad. Add colorful vegetables, too, and fruits if you'd like. Eat as much salad as you want. You won't gain weight by eating salad (unless you drown it in a high-fat dressing). Try fresh-squeezed fruit juices or fat-free organic dressings. Strive to eat at least a pound of raw greens a day.

Eat fresh fruit at least three times a day. If you normally eat sweets at night, eat a sweet fruit at night; it will satisfy your sweet tooth, and fruit is packed with antioxidants. Eat more fruit if you'd like, but try not to eat too many fruits with low nutrient densities.

Explore new fruits and vegetables in your grocery store. Better yet, explore new grocery stores and farmer's markets. When's the last time you ate kale, bok choy, or kiwi? Buy a variety of fruits and vegetables. You'll soon discover that you were missing out by eating the same processed foods week after week, and you'll have fun trying new, healthy recipes.

If you live in a suitable climate, you might enjoy starting your own vegetable garden in your back patio. A little garden that's only about 10 square-feet provides plenty of tomatoes, peppers, onions, collards, squash, and melons.

You might also want to plant an herb garden. Herbs are easy to grow, and you can even grow them indoors. Fresh herbs add flavor and nutrients to any dish.

Limit starchy vegetables and whole grains to one cup a day. Starchy vegetables like squash, carrots, and potatoes are much healthier than starchy grains like rice. When you must have grains, choose unrefined grains brown rice or wild rice, and restrict portion sizes. I have a bowl of natural steel-cut oatmeal for breakfast once every couple of weeks, but I know that I cannot eat grains for breakfast every day.

Try to eat at a cup of beans a day. They have high nutrient densities, and they go well with vegetables. Beans will help you fill you up. Add some beans to your cooked greens or to your salad. On the weekend, you can make enough bean soup to last throughout the week.

Limit your consumption of nuts and seeds to one handful a day. They're healthy and high in nutrients but also high in calories. Many of my patients sprinkle flaxseed on their salads; flaxseed is a great source of omega-3 fat.

In Eat to Live, Dr. Fuhrman recommends that you keep things simple. Don't give yourself an excuse to go out for fast food or call for delivery! Dr. Fuhrman's sample meal plan for his cleansing diet includes fresh fruit for breakfast; salad, beans, and fruit for lunch; and salad and two cooked vegetables for dinner, followed by a fruit dessert. Of course, if you eat meat, you can also have a small serving of organic, lean meat at dinner – but keep the portion small.

The key to sticking with a healthy, whole food diet is to not let yourself get hungry. Most diets fail because people get hungry and return to old habits and comfort foods. Stuff yourself with salad and cooked greens. If you know you're going out to eat, eat an apple or a salad beforehand, and you won't order as much food at the restaurant.

The Skinny on Fats

Of the three energy producing macronutrients (protein, carbs, and fat), fat is the one that's most likely to contribute to weight gain. The body must expend energy and burn calories in order to store proteins and carbs as fat; however, fat is already fat, so it takes a minimal amount of energy to store it as fat. As a matter of fact, surgeons can extract fat tissue from the body and tell us whether it came from chicken fat, olive oil, vegetable oil, or another source of fat!

Furthermore, fat contains more energy than protein and carbs. In other words, fat is more fattening. All fats contain nine calories per gram, while protein and carbs contain four calories per gram.

But not all fats are created equal (and not all fats are bad). Our body needs a healthy amount of fat. Essential fatty acids, for example, aid in growth and development as well as the prevention of disease. We have to consume essential fatty acids in our diet because the body cannot manufacture them.

The two main essential fatty acids are lenoleic acids and alpha-linolenic acids. Lenoleic acids are omega-6 fats that form arachidonic acid in the body. Over consumption of arachidonic acid promotes inflammation that's associated with high blood pressure, arthritis, and other diseases.

Alpha-lenolenic acids are omega-3 fats that form docosahexainoic acid (DHA) in the body. DHA promotes the production of anti-inflammatory chemicals. Studies show that high levels of arachidonic acid and low levels of omega-3 fats can contribute to heart disease, depression, and increased cancer risk, among other diseases.

Most Americans consume too many omega-6 fats (from processed foods and refined vegetable oils) and not enough omega-3 fats. Walnuts, flaxseed, and cold-water fish like salmon and sardines are good sources of omega-3 fats. Avoid processed foods and sprinkle ground flaxseed on your salad to balance your fats and eliminate inflammation.

You should also avoid consuming too many saturated fats found in meat, eggs, and dairy. Excess consumption of saturated fats is associated with heart disease.

Hydrogenated fats are synthetic fats that utilize trans fatty acids to extend the shelf life or products like margarine. Hydrogenated fats are common in processed food, and you should avoid them whenever possible.

Polyunsaturated fat includes corn oil, soybean oil, and safflower oil. These refined fats promote inflammation and should be avoided. Unsaturated fat is a combination of polysaturated and monosaturated fat, and you should minimize your intake of unsaturated fat.

Monosaturated fats are found in olive oil, avocados, almonds, and most nuts and seeds. Monosaturated fats are healthier than other types of fats, but if you want to lose weight, you should avoid all excess fat in your diet. If you're overweight, then your body already has plenty of fat stored up, and you don't need fat in your diet.

You Are What You Drink

Water may be considered the fourth macronutrient. While you can survive for several weeks without food, you can only survive for a few days without water. The body is 72 percent water, and it's necessary for flushing out toxins and waste.

If you're trying to lose weight, you should drink at least eight tall glasses of water a day. When you don't drink enough clean water, your kidneys cannot properly perform their job of filtering waste and toxins – and part of their workload gets dumped on the liver. This interferes with the liver's ability to metabolize fat stored in the body.

When you drink enough water (at least eight tall glasses a day), then your liver can metabolize fat much faster, and your intestines can absorb nutrients more efficiently, which helps to eliminate food cravings. The result is natural, healthy weight loss.

Adequate water consumption is also the best way to reduce water retention. When you don't drink enough water, your body perceives this shortage as a threat and therefore retains more water, which causes swelling, bloating, and weight gain.

Dr. Melina Jampolis of CNN.com recently reported on a study which showed that people who drink two glasses of water 20 to 30 minutes before every meal lose weight more quickly and lose more weight than those who don't. There you have it! Drink two glasses of purified water before each meal to aid in weight loss.

Be sure to drink purified water. Tap water or even bottled water may contribute to your body's toxic load. You can find a quality home water purifier for under a hundred bucks. See www.AmbrosiaWaterFilters.com for several different options.

Choose Organic Foods Whenever Possible

By choosing organic foods, you will avoid ingesting genetically modified organisms, chemical fertilizers and pesticides, and other synthetic ingredients. Furthermore, several studies show that organic foods offer more nutrients and health benefits than their contaminated counterparts.

An extensive European study found that organic fruits and vegetables contain up to 40 percent more antioxidants. The study also found that organic milk had up to 90 percent more antioxidants.

A recent Australian study found that organically grown kiwis have higher levels of vitamin C and antioxidants. Since organic food supplies more nutrients and does not contribute to your toxic load, it can certainly help you lose weight faster.

I know that organic food is more expensive, and I know you can't buy organic all the time. But it's important to buy the organic versions of certain foods as often as possible. Meat, for example, tends to have the highest levels of pesticides (since it's higher up on the food chain). When it comes to meat, dairy, eggs, berries, and lettuce, try to only buy organic. According to *Consumer Reports,* you should try to buy the organic varieties of the following foods whenever possible: Apples, baby food, bell peppers, celery, cherries, dairy, eggs, imported grapes, meat, nectarines, peaches, pears, poultry, potatoes, red raspberries, spinach, and strawberries.

What Happens When I Mess Up?

Most people can't eat healthy all the time. In our fast food society, sometimes junk food is the only food available. I try to eat healthy 90 percent of the time, and I allow myself to eat junk food (or less-than-ideal food) 10 percent of the time.

I also weigh myself (and my patients) each week. Whenever I gain weight, I go on a mini-cleanse to flush out toxins and lose the extra weight. When you mess up, don't give up hope. Cleanse your body, flush out those toxins, and go back to healthy habits. This is how you will achieve permanent weight loss.

God's Diet Plan: Natural Foods

Once you look at all the research, it becomes clear that God had the perfect diet plan for us all along. If you eat unrefined, natural foods and avoid processed foods, then you will not only lose weight but also balance your pH level, balance your omega-3 and omega-6 fats, and deflame your body. God intended for us to eat whole vegetables and fruits, raw nuts and seeds, beans, and lean meats. God never intended for us to start producing food like it's an industrial product.

In evolutionary terms, the human body is not equipped to digest toxic food additives and the most inflammatory foods like refined grains and dairy products. When you think about it, isn't it a little odd that we humans drink so much cow's milk? That milk was made for baby cows, not for humans! Indeed, many experts believe that humans should not drink milk past infancy. Dr. Frank Oski, Director of Pediatrics at Johns Hopkins School of Medicine, says, "No one should drink milk."

It appears that most of the world agrees with Dr. Oski. More than 70 percent of the world's population does not drink milk! The United States has only 4 percent of the world's population but consumes more dairy than the other 96 percent of the planet's population.

Milk is promoted as a good way to prevent osteoporosis because of its relatively high calcium content; however, the animal protein in milk also intensifies the urinary excretion of calcium and may increase the risk of bone fractures. If milk were really good for our bones, the United States would have the strongest bones in the world. Instead, we have one of the highest rates of osteoporosis in the world! Vegetables like broccoli, chard, and kale are rich sources of calcium. We humans should be getting our calcium from the same place cows get theirs - from plants. Our bodies are simply not equipped to digest so much milk from another species.

Our bodies are not equipped to digest grains, either. Our bodies are designed to eat the natural foods of a hunter-gatherer society. Dr. Loren Cordain, PhD, author of *The Paleo Diet*, explains that a mere 500 generations ago, before the agricultural revolution took hold and people started growing cereal grains and domesticating cows, our ancestors ate fresh fruits and vegetables, nuts and seeds, and lean meats. (Inflammatory corn-fed beef didn't exist back then!)

"On a calorie-by-calorie basis, whole grains are lousy sources of fiber, minerals, and B vitamins when compared to the lean meats, seafood, and fresh fruit and veggies that dominate The Paleo Diet," writes Dr. Cordain. "For example, a 1,000-calorie serving of fresh fruits and vegetables has between two and seven times as much fiber as does a comparable serving of whole grains. In fruits and veggies most of the fiber is heart-healthy, soluble fiber that lowers cholesterol levels -- the same cannot be said for the insoluble fiber that is predominant in most whole grains. A 1,000-calorie serving of whole grain cereal contains 15 times less calcium, three times less magnesium, 12 times less potassium, six times less iron, and two times less copper than a comparable serving of fresh vegetables. Moreover, whole grains contain a substance called phytate that almost entirely prevents the absorption of any calcium, iron, or zinc that is found in whole grains, whereas the type of iron, zinc, and copper found in lean meats and seafood is in a form that is highly absorbed."

It's no wonder that so many people have trouble digesting dairy and refined grains. They're not the foods that God intended for us to eat, and our bodies cannot properly assimilate their nutrients. God intended for us to eat fresh fruits and vegetables, nuts, seeds, beans, and lean meats. Follow God's diet plan, and you will receive many blessings in the way of health.

Try to practice mindful eating. Be aware of what you're eating and how you're eating it. Be aware of how the food was prepared. Before you order a meal in a restaurant or fill up your plate at home, ask yourself if the food you're going to put on your plate will heal you or harm you. Is it inflammatory or anti-inflammatory? Is it acid-forming or alkalizing? Is it processed or natural?

Before you eat a meal, drink a glass of purified water. When you sit down to a meal, eat slowly and mindfully. If you eat too quickly, you won't notice when your body is full. Pay attention to your body's signals. When you feel full, stop eating. Drink some more water, or have a little fruit for dessert.

Think about your food; think about where it came from and what kind of effects it will have on your body. Enjoy your food – relish the various flavors – but do not allow yourself to become emotionally attached to your food. You should seek emotional fulfillment from other people, not from food (no matter what those fast food commercials would have us believe).

Let food be your medicine.

{ "Mother Nature is an infinitely more ingenious and exciting chemist."

-Leslie Taylor }

7

The Healing Power of Plants

Plants are nature's pharmacy. There are hundreds of examples of the medicinal benefits of plants. They have contributed to the healing of many diseases. In fact, true healing of any illness comes from within the body, from a healing response initiated by healthy immune system function. God designed our body to heal itself. If you cut your finger your body immediately begins the process of mending and healing the wound. This is a natural response and works well if the body's healing system is healthy and intact. A healthy immune system requires proper nutrition to remain at its optimal function. There are many stories of people who have restored their health by giving their body the nutrients it was deficient in through plant based nutrition. One such story is told by Leslie Taylor. In her mid-20s, Leslie Taylor survived a rare form of leukemia by turning to herbal medicine. She has been researching the healing power of plants ever since.

When Leslie heard that a rainforest herb known as "cat's claw" was being used to treat cancer and AIDS in Europe, she reviewed the research and boarded a plane to Peru.

After learning more about the medicinal plant, Leslie had a vision of making cat's claw available in the United States as a natural supplement.

"Not only did I find this vine called cat's claw growing in the rainforest," writes Leslie on her homepage, leslietaylor.com, "I found a wealth of medicinal plants growing in an incredible environment that were more effective than any I've seen. I fell in love with the wildness of the jungles, the innocence and spirit of the native peoples, the vast and varied cultures, and the spirit, energy and power of the rainforest."

Recent research shows that phytochemicals in cat's claw appear to act as anti-inflammatory, antioxidant, antiviral, antibacterial, immunostimulant, and anticancer agents. (Phyto comes from a Greek word meaning plant.) While our society only recently learned of cat's claw, it has been used by the indigenous peoples of South and Central America for at least 2,000 years.

The practice of using medicinal plants dates back to prehistoric times. The Lascaux cave paintings in France, some of which are dated at 30,000 years old, appear to depict the use of plants as healing agents.

The earliest healers probably discovered medicinal plants by closely observing nature. When they get sick, many animals can be seen eating bitter herbs that they would normally avoid. Sick animals tend to seek out bitter plants that are rich in phytochemicals like tannins and alkaloids. Many phytochemicals are secondary metabolites; that is, they are not necessary to the functioning of the plants, but they often help the plant defend itself or disperse its seeds.

Many phytochemicals give plants their distinctive colors. Phytochemicals called carotenoids include yellow, orange, and red pigments found in fruits and vegetables. Leafy green vegetables are actually rich in the carotenoids, but the yellow pigmentation is masked by the green chloraphyll that's abundant in leaves. Flavonoids produce reddish pigments, like those in grape skins.

Phytochemicals are also referred to as phytonutrients, although this term is somewhat of a misnomer since phytonutrients don't provide nutritional value in the conventional sense. They do, however, offer many health benefits.

Alkaloids, the most common type of secondary metabolites found in plants, are naturally occurring organic compounds produced by many organisms, including bacteria, fungi, plants, and animals, and many of them are used as stimulants or anesthetics. Alkaloids appear in 45 percent of tropical plants. Cocaine, opium, nicotine, caffeine, dopamine, and serotonin are all alkaloid chemicals. In nature, nicotine serves as a natural pesticide for the plants that produce it. Plants that contain alkaloids tend to have a bitter taste.

Plants containing tannins are usually bitter, too. Tannins belong to a group of phytochemicals known as polyphenols, many of which act as antioxidants. Tea, wine, and most berries contain tannins.

Luckily for us, we don't have to journey to jungles of Peru or purchase an obscure supplement to enjoy the health benefits of phytochemicals. All you have to do is eat your fruits and veggies! Flavonoids, for example, can be found in all citrus fruits, berries, onions, parsley, tea, and dark chocolate. Flavonoids, like tannins, are polyphenols, and many flavonoids promote antioxidant activity in the body. Flavonoids offer anti-inflammatory, anti-microbial, and anti-cancer benefits.

UCLA cancer researchers found that people who ate foods containing certain flavonoids were protected from lung cancer. Dr. Zuo-Feng Zhang of UCLA's Jonsson Cancer Center said that the most protective flavonoids appear to be catechin, found in strawberries and tea; kaempferol, found in brussel sprouts and apples; and quercetin, found in beans, onions, and apples.

Here's a brief list of some common phytonutrients along with some of the foods that supply them:

Carotenoids

Alpha-carotene - carrots
Beta-carotene - leafy green and deep yellow vegetables (kale, broccoli, sweet potato, pumpkin)
Beta-cryptoxanthin - apricots, peaches, citrus fruits
Lutein - leafy greens like spinach, collards, and kale
Lycopene - tomato products, pink grapefruit, watermelon
Zeaxanthin - green vegetables, citrus fruits

Flavonoids

Anthocyanins - various fruits
Catechins - tea, wine
Flavonines - citrus fruits
Flavones - various fruits and vegetables
Flavonols - fruits, vegetables, tea, wine
Isoflavones - soybeans, lentils, peanuts
Besides carotenoids and flavonoids, other phytonutrients include inositol phosphates (phytates), lignans, isothiocyanates, phenols, saponins, sulfides, and terpenes.

Forgotten Roots

Less than two hundred years ago, virtually all medicines were plant-based. John Rudolphy's *Pharmaceutical Directory of All the Crude Drugs Now in General Use,* published in 1872, lists all medicinal plants known to treat illnesses. At that time, few synthetic chemicals were used in pharmacies. Synthetic chemicals didn't become widespread in medicine until the early 1990s, and World War II ushered in a plethora of new synthetic chemicals. Even today, 37 percent of prescribed medicines in the United States have active ingredients that are derived from rainforest plants.[6]

Yet somehow, as the modern age took hold, the entire modern medical establishment seemed to forget medicine's natural roots. Pharmaceuticals were synthesized in laboratories, not harvested from jungles or fields. As a society, we forgot our place in nature. The chemical revolution affected the food industry, too. Food became an engineered product rather than a natural gift from God. Pharmaceutical companies took over medical schools, and medical schools stopped teaching their students about the healing power of plants. Instead, they taught future doctors how to write prescriptions and turn profits. Somehow, the foundation of modern medicine had become relegated to "alternative" medicine.

Only a few years ago, herbalism was considered to be alternative medicine, scoffed at as quackery by many medical doctors. But, now modern science is showing that natural healers are in fact highly effective. In their embrace of herbalism medical researchers typically refer to the study of medicinal plant-based chemicals as phytotherapy rather than herbalism. And "phytotherapy" is one hot buzzword in scientific circles! From 1997 to 2007, the number of research papers listed on PubMed containing the word "phytotherapy" grew from less than 1,000 to more than 15,000. (PubMed is a service of the US National Library of Medicine that archives biomedical research articles.)

Here's the thing about herbal extracts: many beneficial phytochemicals lose much of their potency once they're extracted. Herbal extracts are processed plant materials. Like processed foods, processed herbs can lose their intrinsic value during the "processing" process. Many phytochemicals need to be in the presence of specific enzymes and cofactors in order to perform their natural functions.

An enzyme is a bimolecule (usually a protein) that initiates or speeds up a chemical reaction. For example, our saliva contains enzymes that begin the process of digestion before food is even swallowed. Many enzymes require cofactors, or helper molecules, to assist in biochemical reactions. Vitamins and minerals often play the role of cofactors.

Scientists are only beginning to understand the complex chemistry involved in phytochemical reactions; thousands of phytochemicals have yet to be discovered. But one thing's for sure: Mother Nature is an infinitely more exciting and ingenious chemist than the scientists employed by pharmaceutical and agricultural laboratories!

Since plants lose much of their healing power when they're processed, it's important to eat whole foods in their natural state. Refined foods offer empty calories without the natural health benefits inherent in plants. Whole foods come complete with their own enzymes and cofactors. Plant enzymes include cellulose (which digests fiber), lipase (which digests fat), amylase (which digests carbohydrates), and protease (which digests protein).

"Unfortunately, in America and other Westernized countries, most people do not eat whole foods, and those who do have trouble digesting them because most foods are eaten cooked and have zero enzymes," explains Dr. Lita Lee, PhD, author of *The Enzyme Cure*. "Thus, the need for whole foods and enzyme nutrition is widespread . . . People think that if they simply take vitamins and minerals they will be healthy, but every vitamin and mineral requires an enzyme. You can eat pounds and pounds of vitamins and minerals, but if you don't have the proper enzymes, they don't work."

Plant enzymes not only aid in the digestion of food, but they also assist the immune system in digesting and eliminating toxins. Some enzymes, for example, digest the coating on viruses, allowing the immune system to destroy the virus.

When you eat unrefined plant foods with their natural enzymes and cofactors intact, the phytonutrients can do their job. Some phytonutrients serve as cofactors to activate enzymes produced by the body. Different phytonutrients may act as antioxidants, enhance immune function, repair DNA damage, kill cancer cells, and detoxify carcinogens. Countless medical studies prove that eating fruits and vegetables will make your healthier and reduce your risk of disease. Here are some highlights from medical research journals:

Fruit and vegetable consumption has been linked to a

decreased risk of stroke. Three daily servings of fruits and vegetables lower the risk of stroke by 22 percent. Imagine what six servings can do!

Men who eat at least two servings of dark green or deep yellow vegetables a day have a 46 percent decrease in heart disease risk and a 70 percent decrease in cancer risk compared to those who consume less than one serving daily. This study shows that very small changes in your eating habits - eating a couple of salads a day - can go a long way in preventing the most deadly diseases in our society.

Consumption of tomato products have been linked to a decreased risk of prostate cancer. Men who consume 10 or more servings a week of tomato products have a 35% lower chance of prostate cancer compared to those who eat 1.5 or fewer servings per week. Ten servings may sound like a lot, but if you're eating a couple of salads a day and adding a sliced tomato to each salad, it's easy to get those 10 servings. Note that processed ketchup will not provide the same benefits as a whole tomato, not to mention ketchup is loaded with refined sugar! A single tomato contains thousands of different phytonutrients.

Another study found that men who eat three or more servings of cruciferous vegetables a week have a 41 percent decreased rate of prostate cancer. Cruciferous vegetables like cabbage and broccoli are high in isothiocyanates, which activate enzymes that detoxify carcinogens.

People who eat a lot of spinach or collards (both high in lutein), have a 46 percent decrease in the risk of age-related macular degeneration compared to those who consume greens less than once a month. Eat your greens if you appreciate your eyesight!

America's Top Two Killers

Cancer and heart disease, America's top two killers, are such scary, devastating diseases, not only for victims, but also for family members and friends. Why are cancer and heart disease so prevalent in our society? For one thing, most Americans are simply not eating enough vegetables. Typical Americans get 42 percent of their calories from animal foods and 51 percent of their calories from refined carbohydrates and oils.

"The most compelling evidence of the last decade has indicated the importance of protective factors, largely unidentified, in fruits and vegetables," said Walter Willett, MD, PhD, who spoke before the American Association for Cancer Research.

In *Eat to Live,* Dr. Fuhrman lists five ways that phytochemicals prevent cancer:

1. *Phytochemicals detoxify and deactivate cancer-causing agents and block the initiation process leading to DNA damage.*
2. *Phytochemicals fuel cellular mechanisms to repair damaged DNA sequences, bringing the cell back to normal.*
3. *Phytochemicals impede proliferation or duplication of cells with DNA damage.*
4. *Phytochemicals protect the DNA against further damage.*
5. *Phytochemicals inhibit the spread of cancerous cells.*

If you want to protect yourself against cancer, you should be eating a wide variety of vegetables every day. Raw vegetables are the best cancer fighters. Add plenty of raw veggies to your salads. If you follow the diet plan outlined in Chapter 6 and get most of your calories from whole foods with high nutrient densities, then you'll get plenty of cancer-fighting phytonutrients.

Let's take a look at just some of the phytonutrients in a few foods with high nutrient densities:

Kale: The organosulfur compounds in kale have been a prominent subject among phytotherapy researchers. Organosulfur compounds in kale include glucosinolates and methyl cysteine sulfoxides. Both of these phytonutrients activate detoxifying enzymes in the liver that help neutralize carcinogens. Sulforaphane, for instance, is a powerful glucosinolate that allows the liver to eliminate carcinogens more efficiently by enhancing enzyme activity. Sulforaphane is formed when you chew kale. In animal studies, it has been shown to inhibit chemically-induced breast cancers and destroy colon cancer cells by altering the expression of cancer related genes.

Dr. Tony Kong of Rutgers University, who studied the cancer-fighting ability of sulforaphane, said, "Our study corroborates the notion that sulforaphne has chemo protective activity . . . Our research has substantiated the connection between diet and cancer prevention, and it is now clear that the expression of cancer-related genes can be influenced by chemo preventive compounds in the things we eat."

Several studies show that cruciferous vegetables like kale, cabbage, cauliflower, and broccoli offer significant protection against lung cancer, colon cancer, breast cancer, and ovarian cancer. A recent University of Texas study found that they also offer protection against bladder cancer; study participants who ate the most cruciferous vegetables had a 29 percent lower risk of bladder cancer. The anti-cancer benefits of phytonutrients in cruciferous vegetables are even more pronounced for those groups who are at high risk for developing bladder cancer: men, smokers (current and former), and individuals older than 64.

In fact, cruciferous vegetables appear to be better cancer fighters than other types of vegetables. The ongoing Netherlands Cohort Study on Diet and Cancer found that people eating the most vegetables had a 25 percent lower risk of colorectal cancer - but those eating the most cruciferous vegetables had 49 percent decrease in colorectal cancer risk. Another Chinese study found that regular consumption of cruciferous vegetables reduced the risk of lung cancer among smokers by an amazing 69 percent!

Kale also supplies a flavonoid called kaempferol. A major Nurses' Health Study conducted between 1984 and 2002 revealed that women whose diets were high in kaempferol enjoyed a 40 percent risk in the reduction of ovarian cancer, compared to women who ate few foods with kaempferol. Other foods containing kaempferol include broccoli, leeks, spinach, and blueberries. (Note that they're all foods with high nutrient densities!)

For several years, scientists have known that many phytonutrients act as antioxidants, sweeping up free radicals before they damage DNA. But researchers have only recently discovered that phytonutrients in cruciferous vegetables like kale work on a much deeper level - by actually altering the expression of genes. For example, some phytochemicals signal our genes to produce more helpful enzymes that cleanse the body of toxins.

Kale also provides carotenoids like lutein and zeaxanthin, which keep the eyes healthy, as well as indole-3-carbinol (I-3-C), a metabolite of glucosinate phytonutrients that lowers levels of LDL cholesterol. One study found that liver cells treated with I-3-C cut their production of a particular LDL transporter protein in half. The study also found that I-3-C lowered triglyceride levels.

Now would be a good time to lightly steam some kale. Collards and other crucifers offer many of the same phytonutrients. Buy organic greens and lightly steam them to get the most out of your phytonutrients.

Romaine Lettuce: Romaine lettuce is rich in vitamin C and the phytonutrient beta-carotene. These two nutrients work together to prevent the oxidation of cholesterol. When cholesterol is oxidized, it becomes sticky and can build up on arterial walls, forming plaques that cause heart disease. It's interesting to note that some studies show that beta-carotene supplements do not provide the same heart healthy effects as beta-carotene from whole plants. Once again, we see that God had a perfect diet plan all along and Mother Nature is the wisest chemist of all.

Bell Peppers: These sweet peppers are among a select group of vegetables that provide lycopene, a carotenoid that provides protection against cancers of the prostate, cervix, bladder, and pancreas.

Bell peppers also contain beta-cryptoxanthin, an orange-red carotenoid also found in pumpkin, papaya, tangerines, peaches, and organes. This phytonutrient may significantly lower your risk of lung cancer. One study of 60,000 adults found that those eating the most cryptoxanthin-rich foods had a 27 percent reduction in lung cancer risk. The study also found that smokers who ate the most cryptoxanthin-rich foods had a 37 percent risk of lung cancer compared to smokers who ate few foods containing bea-cryptoxanthin.

Tomatoes: Lycopene is also found in tomatoes, as well as carotenoids and beta-carotene. It's not just the lycopene in tomatoes that protects against cancer and heart disease; rather, it's the synergy of the thousands of phytonutrients in tomatoes that work together. Even ketchup, tomato sauce, and tomato juice provide antioxidant activity. Of course, the natural, organic versions of these products are much healthier. A USDA study found that organic ketchup contains three times the amount of lycopene. Now, tomato sauce may be healthy, but that doesn't mean that you should eat pasta or pizza every day. Add tomato sauce and Italian herbs to beans and wild rice for a tasty, healthier alternative to pasta.

One study found that broccoli and tomatoes eaten together combine to provide strong anti-cancer protection. A diet rich in broccoli and tomatoes was found to shrink cancerous prostate tumors more than a diet rich in one vegetable or the other.

"When tomatoes and broccoli are eaten together, we see an additive effect. We think it's because different bioactive compounds in each food work on different anti-cancer pathways," said Professor John Erdman of the University of Illinois.

"Older men with slow-growing prostate cancer who have chosen watchful waiting over chemotherapy and radiation should seriously consider altering their diets to include more tomatoes and broccoli," reported Kirstie Canene-

Adams, a fellow researcher.

Sea Vegetables: Sea vegetables (also known as seaweed) contain phytonutrients called lignans that inhibit tumor growth. Flaxseed also contains lignans. Some types of seaweed also contain unique polysaccharides known as fucans, which reduce the level of inflammation in the body.

Blueberries: These small berries not only taste great, but they're packed with anthocyanins. Anthocyanins are phytonutrients with blue-red pigmentation that appear to enhance the structural integrity of blood vessels. One study found that anthocyanins also enhance memory and learning ability and may reduce the chance of neurodegenerative diseases like Alzheimer's. Another study shows that anthocyanins and other phytonutrients in blueberries inhibit cancer cell proliferation. But blueberry pie doesn't offer the same health benefits. Research reveals that canned foods and processed foods made from blueberries contained virtually no anthocyanins. You've got to eat the whole food if you want the health benefits.

Humans have been eating unrefined plant foods for thousands of years. Our bodies need phytonutrients in order to work properly; our bodies depend on these chemicals which have co-evolved with the chemicals in our bodies. Unfortunately, the typical American diet, in which most calories come from animal foods and processed foods, does not provide an adequate supply of phytonutrients. You can't pour sugar water in a gasoline tank and expect the engine to turn over, and you can't dump toxic, processed food into your body on an ongoing basis and expect it to keep running smoothly. Eventually, the machinery will break down on a cellular level.

A Note on Animal Proteins

I am not a vegetarian or an anti-meat crusader by any means. I love to eat a nice steak occasionally. But I cannot ignore the research which shows that too much animal protein has toxic effects on the body.

In *Eat to Live,* Dr. Furhman points out that animal protein raises cholesterol, promotes cancer, promotes bone loss, promotes kidney disease, accelerates aging, and comes packaged with saturated fat, cholesterol, and acrachidonic acid. Plant protein, on the other hand, lowers cholesterol, protects against cancer, promotes bone strength, and comes packaged with fiber, antioxidants, and phtyonutrients. The China Project, which is probably the largest epidemiological study ever done on the relationship between diet and the risk of disease, showed that cancer and heart disease increase as consumption of animal food increases.

Because the United States Department of Agriculture promotes animal products so heavily, there are many common misconceptions about animal protein. Patients often ask, "Don't I need to eat meat to get enough protein?"

I reply with a question of my own: "Well, let me ask you this, which food has more protein - steak or broccoli?" Invariably, most people think that steak contains more protein - but, in fact, steak has only 5.4 grams of protein per 100 calories while broccoli has 11.2 grams. Broccoli contains almost twice as much protein as steak on a per-calorie basis! Vegetarians who eat a variety of vegetables, beans, nuts, and seeds get plenty of amino acids and proteins in their diet.

With that said, I don't ask my patients to become vegans or vegetarians. Instead, I ask them to limit their intake of meat - and when they do eat meat, it should be lean, organic, free-range meat. And I try to practice what I preach (except when I'm in Chicago and there's Ginno's Pizza!). I'm planning to live a long, healthy life. In accordance, I eat my vegetables every day.

I know that health doesn't come from a pill bottle. Health comes from a diet rich in unrefined, whole plants foods, healthy movement on a regular basis, and a healthy state of mind.

> "The second day of a diet is always easier than the first, By the second day, you're off it."
> — Jackie Gleason

8

Why Fad Diets Don't Work

From the Atkins diet to the grapefruit diet (and everything in between), fad diets simply don't work. Many fad diets will help you lose weight temporarily, but once you go off the diet, the weight will come back. Plus, many fad diets will leave you less healthy than you were before you started the diet.

To lose weight and get healthy, you must eat plenty of whole, unrefined foods with high nutrient densities and avoid processed foods with low nutrient densities. **Don't allow yourself to get hungry!** Stuff yourself with salads. When you get hungry, eat - but eat right.

The Problem with Calorie Restriction Diets

The traditional diet plan for weight loss revolves around calorie restriction. Eat what you want, it recommends, but count the calories and make sure that you have a calorie deficit. As long as you're burning more calories than you consume, then you'll lose weight.

My first diet was the grapefruit diet. By eating a grapefruit before every meal, I ate smaller amounts of high-calorie foods. As a Fat Boy, I was so motivated to lose weight that I sometimes skipped meals. The problem was that I eventually got hungry. I'd slip back into old habits and regain the weight. Over the years, I slowly put on more weight. My cycle of yo-yo dieting continued for many years, throughout many different fad diets.

Diet programs like Jenny Craig and NutriSystem supply prepackaged, low-calorie processed meals. I shudder every time I see a commercial for one of these programs. People are paying outrageous amounts of money to eat nothing but fake food packaged in packaging that adds to its toxicity. Eventually, people on calorie-restriction diets get hungry and go off the diet. Or they lose a few pounds, go off the diet, and gain back the weight plus some.

Calorie restriction diets don't work because people get hungry - especially when they eat nothing but microwave meals low in nutrition. That's just not healthy! They're missing out on healthy nutrients and enzymes. Thus, they never feel satisfied.

Atkins Insanity

Looking back, I can't believe that I actually taught classes on the Atkins diet. What was I thinking? I was probably thinking, "Hey, now here's a diet that I can live with." I was addicted to food, and this diet allowed me to have all the steak, bacon, eggs, and butter that I wanted. All I had to do was stay away from those pesky fruits and vegetables, which were loaded with carbs. As a food addict, how could I not love this diet? I could eat all the high-protein, high-fat foods that I wanted and still lose weight. It was amazing!

I remember salivating as I read the first page of *Dr. Atkins Health Revolution*:

Imagine losing weight with a diet that lets you have bacon and eggs for breakfast, heavy cream in your coffee, plenty of meat and even salad with dressing for lunch and dinner!

A food addict's fantasy! Little did I know, this fantasy can easily turn into a health nightmare.

Here's how the high-protein, low-carb diets work: You're

allowed to eat all the meat, cheese, and fat that you want, but you have to keep your consumption of carbs very low. This means no pasta, no starchy vegetables, no whole grains, and very little fruit. By strictly avoiding carbohydrates, you trigger a survival mechanism known as ketogensis, which puts your body in a state of ketosis. When you don't eat carbohydrates, your body breaks fatty acids down into ketones, an emergency fuel supply. Ketosis allows your body to survive without breaking down muscle tissue. But as soon as you start eating carbs again, your metabolism will return to normal, and you will gain weight, especially if you're still eating steak, bacon, eggs, and butter every day.

Ketosis is not a normal, healthy state for the body. It is a crisis state that should be reserved for true emergencies. The metabolism of so much protein puts extra stress on the liver and kidneys. A high-protein diet causes the kidneys to age prematurely. Diabetics are particularly sensitive to the effects of a high-protein diet. One study found that many diabetics who ate too much animal protein lost over half of their kidney function, and most of the damage was permanent.

Low-carb, high-protein diets like the Atkins diet may cause permanent liver and kidney damage, osteoporosis (since animal protein promotes the loss of calcium through the urine), kidney stones, high cholesterol, and cancer, among other health problems. The Atkins diet causes problems on one level because of too much animal protein, and it causes problems on another level because you're not getting the health benefits of plant substances like vitamins, minerals, fiber, and phytochemicals.

A friend of mine who tried the Atkins diet had a bad habit of forgetting to take her daily multi-vitamin. She began losing her hair. Actually, the majority of her hair fell out! She went back to eating carbs (healthy carbs this time), and her hair grew back. Could there be a correlation? You bet! I blamed my friend for not taking her vitamins, not the diet itself for being incomplete. I continued teaching the

Atkins diet and enjoying my steaks, not truly aware of the damage that I was doing to my body.

Well, I wasn't totally unaware. I knew that something wasn't quite right (but I was really enjoying those steaks). The diet caused bad breath, headaches, nausea, and constipation. These were signs that I wasn't healthy. In my mind, I justified my symptoms as sacrifices. *No pain, no gain,* right?

My wallet was feeling the pain, too. I had to spend a lot of money on supplements. As we've seen, supplements simply don't provide the same health benefits as whole foods.

I'm very lucky that my daughter introduced me to Dr. Furhman's work. In *Eat to Live,* Dr. Fuhrman reminds us that a diet high in meat increase cancer risk, while diets high in fruits and vegetables decrease cancer risk. A low-carb, high-protein diet causes the body to become acidic, promotes inflammation, and increases the risk of cancer. Following the Atkins diet could more than double your risk of developing certain types of cancer.

Any diet that forbids fruit is unhealthy. Many studies show that there's a strong relationship between fruit consumption and cancer risk. In fact, as Dr. Fuhrman points out, fruit consumption decreases heart disease, cancer, and mortality in general. You must eat a wide variety of fruits and vegetables to maintain good health.

"People need to wake up to the reality that diets that restrict the consumption of entire food groups - especially essential carbohydrates like fruits and vegetables - are unhealthy and can be dangerous," said former U.S. Surgeon General C. Everett Koop.

The Atkins diet plan is nearly the opposite of a healthy, whole food diet. It discourages the consumption of refined sugar, which is great, but it also encourages the over-consumption of animal protein and fats and under-consumption of fruits and vegetables. Moreover, it sets people up to gain more weight as soon as they starting eating carbs again. The Atkins diet allows people to crave high-protein, high-fat foods and satisfy those cravings. As a result, most people end up gaining even more weight in the long-run. And even when they're losing weight, they're setting themselves up for chronic health problems. Other low-carb diets like the South Beach diet may not be quite as unhealthy since they allow for more fruits and vegetables, but they still put a limit on healthy, disease-fighting foods.

The Mediterranean Diet Craze

The Mediterranean diet encourages people to eat plenty of fruits, vegetables, beans, and nuts, but it also encourages the liberal use of olive oil. As far as fats go, olive oil is fine. It's much healthier than butter or corn oil, for instance. But if you want to lose weight, you don't need extra fat in your diet - and olive oil is 100 percent refined fat with a very low nutrient density.

"In the 1950s people living in the Mediterranean, especially on the island of Crete, were lean and virtually free of heart disease. Yet over 40 percent of their caloric intake came from fat, primarily olive oil," notes Dr. Fuhrman in *Eat to Live.* "If we look at the diet they consumed back then, we note that the Cretans ate mostly fruits, vegetables, beans, and some fish. Saturated fat was less than 6 percent of their total fat intake. True, they ate lots of olive oil, but the rest of their diet was exceptionally healthy. They also worked hard in the fields, walking about nine miles a day, often pushing a plow or working other manual farm equipment. Americans didn't take home the message to eat loads of vegetables, beans, and fruits and do loads of exercise; they just accepted that olive oil is a health food.

"Today the people of Crete are fat, just like us. They're still eating a lot of olive oil, but their consumption of fruits, vegetables, and beans is down. Meat, cheese, and fish are their new staples, and their physical activity level has plummeted. Today, heart disease has sky-rocketed and more than half the population of both adults and children in

Crete is overweight."

So much for the Mediterranean diet, unless you implement it as it was prior to 1950.

Stay Out of the Zone

Dr. Fuhram is highly critical of *The Zone* by Barry Sears, PhD. The zone diet is yet another high-protein, high-fat diet. Dr. Sears argues an excess of carbs is behind the obesity epidemic and that people should eat precisely measured portions of the macronutrients (protein, fat, and carbs). According to the zone diet plan, bananas, carrots, and lima beans are off-limits because they have a high glycemic index (which means that the carbohydrates from these foods enter the bloodstream relatively quickly). But a food's glycemic index is not a good indicator of its health value or nutrient density.

"You need not be concerned about the glycemic index of a particular natural food if it is otherwise nutrient- and fiber-rich and is part of a healthful diet," writes Dr. Fuhrman. "In fact, the presence or lack of fiber is a much more reliable predictor of blood glucose control . . . The fiber content of the food or meal is more important than the glycemic index. All these high-protein gurus are forced to neglect the hottest area of nutritional research today - phytochemicals and plant fibers - because it would make their diets look dangerous."

Weight Loss Requires A Lifestyle Change

There are so many other fad diets. I could go over them one by one and explain why they don't work, but I think you get the general idea. Fad diets are unnatural. They don't work because people are either not eating enough food or they're not getting proper nutrition. After a while, they get hungry, go off the diet, and return to previous eating habits. Studies show that dieting alone will not lead to permanent weight loss. In the long-run, nearly all dieters gain back the weight they lost, and about half of them gain back even more weight.

Diets not only make people hungry, but they reduce metabolic rates. When you eat less food, your metabolism slows down. Thus, many people find that, in the long run, they actually gain more weight by dieting. They'll lose 10 pounds, go off the diet, and gain back 15. This is the yo-yo dieting effect.

Yo-yo dieting puts stress on the body. The body strives to maintain homeostasis, or balance, but yo-yo dieting constantly disrupts that homeostasis. Your body's biochemistry has a hard time keeping up with the mixed signals.

One study found that overweight people who have been overweight for most of their lives are actually healthier than people who had lost and gained weight several times. The yo-yo dieters in the study had 30 percent less natural killer cell activity in their immune systems. (Natural killer cells kill viruses and cancer cells.) Before you go on a crash diet, make sure you're ready to lose weight and keep it off by changing your lifestyle.

Lifestyle is key. You cannot expect to lose weight by simply going on a diet. If you want to lose weight, you have to learn how to eat right and change your lifestyle. When you finish reading this book and start your own MET Right program, don't think of it as "going on a diet." Instead, think of the experience as learning how to enjoy a healthy lifestyle. Eating right is only one-third of the weight loss equation. You also have to get moving and change the way you think. When you train yourself to move right, eat right, and think right, then you will lose weight and keep it off. But not until then.

You've learned how to eat right. Now let's learn how to move right and think right.

9

Move Right

According to popular legend, Galileo mumbled "Eppur si mouve!" under his breath after he was found guilty of heresy and forced to recant his theory that the earth revolves around the sun. Eppur si mouve translates to "and yet it moves." Despite recanting his heliocentric theory before the Catholic Inquisition, the father of modern physics spent the remainder of his life under arrest.

"Galileo, perhaps more than any other single person, was responsible for the birth of modern science", writes physicist Stephen Hawking.

Galileo observed that everything in nature is in motion. This is a defining principle of our universe. From the stars in space to the electrons in the atoms that make up our cells, everything is in motion. When applied to a turbine, motion generates energy. When applied to our bodies, motion generates health.

Motion triggers the body's natural repair mechanisms. Where there is motion, there is regeneration; where there is no motion, there is degeneration. In other words, body parts that are not moved frequently begin to die. *Use it or lose it!* Within three days of a lack of movement, body parts begin to degenerate.

Many of my morbidly obese patients have trouble standing, let alone exercising. They don't want to walk, and they don't want to think about putting on a swimsuit and getting in a pool. Exercise can be a real challenge for obese individuals, so I make it as easy as possible. To start moving right, all you have to do is set aside 30 minutes a day to focus on body movement. We don't even have to call it exercise! Let's call in motion therapy. For just 30 minutes a day, engage in some form of movement that goes above and beyond your normal routine. You can do this in the morning before work, in the evening after work, or even during your lunch break.

If you have trouble walking, you can perform your 30 minutes of motion therapy in your chair or even in bed. I refer my patients to HousecallRehab.com, a website that contains flash video tutorials for over 400 stretches and exercises. Many of the movements can be performed while sitting or lying down.

"The first rule of thumb is do no harm," says Dr. Jason Lord, a chiropractor and rehabilitation expert who founded HousecallRehab.com. "A standard exercise program could cause injury or cardiovascular strain to obese individuals. At HousecallRehab.com, the physician can put together a customized plan for the patient and monitor the patient's progress. The site offers low-impact, progressive resistance programs that can be done standing in place, sitting in a chair, or even lying in bed."

I don't care if you sit in your recliner and swing your legs back and forth for 30 minutes - just get moving! Set aside a 30 minutes during the day for your motion therapy; this is your time of healing. Think of your motion therapy as your medicine. It will improve your health much greater than any pill! Spend 40 days turning that 30-minute block of time into a daily habit, and you'll be in shape before you know it.

Don't let television programs like *The Biggest Loser* intimidate you. You don't have to work out two hours a day or hire a personal trainer to lose weight. You just have to get moving and stay moving.

Your motion therapy doesn't have to consist of strenuous activity. In fact, the gentle movements of yoga, tai chi, and qi gong all promote weight loss as well as relaxation (and stress may be preventing you from losing weight, as you'll learn in the next chapter).

Once you feel good enough to get on your feet, find a fun activity that doesn't seem like work. You don't have to *work out*. Get outdoors and play! I joined my church softball league, and it's a blast. I have a lot of fun, and I get in my exercise without even thinking of it as exercise.

If you're up to it, walk for at least a few minutes each day. Walking is a natural body movement that's virtually risk-free in terms of injury. Walk outdoors and you can enjoy the scenery as well as the fresh air and healthy sunlight exposure.

Don't push yourself too hard. Start out slowly, even if you walk only five or ten minutes the first time. Add a few minutes to your walking routine each week, and try to work your way up to 30 minutes. Then start walking faster and trying to get your heart rate up; this will accelerating fat burning and condition your heart and lungs.

Walking will increase your metabolism, improve circulation, stimulate digestion, strengthen and tone your leg muscles, and improve your posture. Focus on your posture when you're walking. Stand up straight and keep your head up. Keep your shoulders held back but relaxed. Pump your arms and breathe deeply to increase the number of calories burned. Keep your strides short and quick, and keep the pace swift. Imagine that you're walking to a beat.

Try to stick with a regular walking routine, whether it's in the morning or in the evening after work. If you normally walk outdoors, have a back-up plan for inclement weather.

If nothing else, you can walk in your local mall. No excuses! Make sure that you wear comfortable, well-fitting sneakers, and drink water before and after you walk. A pedometer will allow you to keep track of the number of steps you take – and it provides a little extra motivation. A walking partner will also provide motivation. (Dogs make great walking partners!)

I've witnessed several patients lose 100 pounds or more by just walking and eliminating junk food from their diet. One gentleman came to see me because he had chronic back pain and heart disease. After I explained the MET Right program to him, he started eating right and walking every morning. He lost 110 pounds in just over a year. He still wakes up at 5:00am every morning to walk. And now he's up to 5 miles a day!

But you don't have to walk 5 miles a day to lose weight. Again, you just have to get moving. Get off the couch and do something, whether it's walking, swimming, bicycling or golfing.

For my more advanced weight loss patients who have been regularly working out for some time, I recommend a combination of aerobic training, strength training, and interval training. Aerobic training includes walking, swimming, and any activity that gets your heart rate up.

Strength training, or weight-bearing exercise, is a highly efficient way to lose weight. Muscle tissue burns calories even when you're sleeping, so the more muscle mass you have, the easier it will be to lose weight. This doesn't mean you have to start pumping iron at the gym or bulk up like the hulk. In fact, you don't even have to lift weights. Walking, for instance, is a weight-bearing exercise as well as an aerobic exercise. Walking will build up your leg muscles and core muscles. Other great body-weight exercises include push-ups, pull-ups, and squats. If you're trying to lose weight, focus on your major muscle groups, especially your legs. Large muscles like those in the legs burn more calories than smaller muscles like those in the arm.

If you decide to start a strength training routine, be sure to give your muscles at least a full day for recovery. On days when you're not building muscle, do some aerobic exercise or interval training.

Interval training is currently very popular among fitness trainers. Sometimes I suggest interval training when advanced patients hit a weight loss plateau. It will kick your metabolism into overdrive. Interval training refers to intense bursts of activity follow by recovery periods of moderate activity.

If you hit a plateau in your walking routine, try intervals of intense speed-walking or jogging. Push yourself hard as hard as you can for one minute, then go back to walking at a moderate pace for three minutes. As your fitness level improves, increase the time of your high intensity intervals. Work toward the goal of jogging for 30 minutes with intervals of sprinting. If you're currently out of shape, this may sound like mission impossible – but it's totally feasible, and it all starts with that first step. Your body has an amazing capacity for change when your mind truly wants it!

When you start doing intervals, you'll probably find that you get tired faster – and that's okay! Since interval training is intense, you won't need to work out as long. The typical interval training session lasts 30 to 45 minutes.

I must warn you: Interval training is intense, and it's not for beginners or morbidly obese individuals (no matter what those television programs would have you believe). Even people who are in good shape should start out with just one or two interval training sessions per week. You have to really push yourself during the intervals to get the benefits. You may find that a training partner helps to motivate you. Over time, as your conditioning improves, increase the difficulty of your intervals. As with strength training, always give your body at least a full day to recover between interval workouts.

You can also do intervals on treadmills, elliptical machines, and stationary bikes. Swimming is a great form of exercise for interval training as well. Since it's difficult (if not impossible) to measure your heart rate with your hand during intense intervals, consider investing in a heart rate monitor; you can get one for about sixty bucks. Work your way up to 30 or 40 minutes of intense interval training per session.

Interval training offers many benefits over traditional endurance training. It burns fat much more efficiently. Interval training primes mitochondria – the little "power stations" in each of your body's cells where fuel is converted into energy – causing them to target fat cells for energy. A recent study in the *Journal of Applied Physiology* showed that just two weeks of interval training increased the amount of fat burned during exercise by 36 percent.

Interval training can improve fitness quickly. Professional athletes have been taking advantage of interval training for decades, but this effective form of exercise has only recently gained mainstream popularity. Athletes and non-athletes alike will tell you that interval training improves fitness quickly – often after just a couple of weeks. One study showed that six out of eight test subjects doubled their endurance after just two weeks of interval training.

Interval training workouts are also much shorter. If you've hit a plateau with walking or jogging, consider interval training. Two hours of interval training per week may produce better results than six hours of jogging per week.

Finally, interval training reduces the risk of injury. Non-stop, long-lasting, repetitive exercises increase the risk of stress injury. Intervals will leave you feeling exhausted, but they don't take long. Note that interval training may increase your appetite. Drink plenty of water before and after your workout to avoid overeating, and if you get hungry, then eat! But choose healthy, whole foods rather than processed foods.

Always check with your healthcare provider before starting any exercise program, especially if you have heart problems. Don't forget to warm up beforehand and cool down afterwards; this will reduce the risk of injury and soreness.

Take your first step today. Before you know it, you'll be out shopping for new clothes to fit your new, slender body.

Chiropractic and Weight Loss

> "The doctor of the future will give no medicine but will interest his patient in the care of the human frame, in diet, and in the cause and prevention of disease."
>
> – Thomas Edison

A chiropractor's primary mission is to care for the frame of the body, particularly the spine and the extremities. A chiropractor checks the structural alignment of the body and looks for places where the motion between joints is restricted or abnormal. Chiropractic adjustments help to restore normal motion.

The spine not only acts as the main support frame for the body but it also protects the spinal cord, the body's main power chord. As part of the central nervous system, the spinal cord extends from the brain and relays electrochemical messages throughout the body. The spinal cord is extremely sensitive - an injury may cause paralysis or death - that is why it's heavily guarded by the bony spine.

The spine is made up of 24 moving bones called vertebrae. When a single vertebra slips out of line or stops moving properly, it can put pressure on the nerves that branch off the spinal cord. Dr. Chung Ha Suh of the University of Colorado showed that a very slight pressure (equal to the weight of a dime) can reduce nerve function by 60 percent. Over time, sustained pressure on a nerve will cause it to deteriorate.

A neural malfunction caused by spinal misalignment

may lead to all sorts of symptoms, including pain, lack of energy, poor immune function, insomnia, indigestion, headaches, allergies, and weight gain. When a spinal misalignment affects the nerve in this manner, the condition is known as a vertebral subluxation. Subluxations may be caused by physical injuries, emotional stress, or biochemical stress. Physical stress may come from sports injuries, auto accidents, or even the birth process. Emotional stress can lead to muscle tension that distorts the spine over time. A poor diet and exposure to toxins may cause biochemical stress and chronic inflammation, which can affect the spine.

Most spinal subluxations get worse over time; this is known as spinal degeneration. When it's caught in time, spinal degeneration can be stopped and reversed. Beyond a certain point, however, the damage is done. It still requires treatment to reduce further degeneration.

A chiropractor is trained to detect and correct spinal problems and reverse or slow the progress of spinal degeneration. By removing the interference from your body's main power cord, chiropractic will not only reduce pain and inflamation but it will also help you achieve holistic health. A healthy spine provides the central communication and control line that the body needs to heal itself.

All of my weight loss patients get regular chiropractic adjustments. The adjustments are like greasing the rusty ball joints on an old car. Adjustments will get the joints moving again. I help patients get moving, and provide them with a stretching and exercise program so they can continue moving at home. This motion will trigger regeneration and healing. Regular chiropractic adjustments are especially important for obese individuals, as the adjustments reduce the risk of stress injuries. The last thing overweight people need is an injury that will prevent them from moving well.

Get Moving and Keep Moving

My kids are lucky. They will never suffer from degenerative joint disease. They have been receiving chiropractic adjustments throughout their lives, and they have been taught to keep moving. Movement promotes healing; a lack of movement promotes disease.

Some medical doctors will tell you that there's no cure for degenerative joint disease, otherwise known as osteoarthritis. They say that it's an age-related disease. If someone goes to a medical doctor with a bad knee, the doctor might say, "There's nothing I can do about it. It's just age."

"Well," the patient might say, "my left knee is just as old as my right knee, and it's fine!"

It is a lack of proper movement that caused degenerative joint disease in the one knee. At some point, some kind of trauma or stress caused that knee to stop moving the way that it should. That stress could've been from a car wreck or from simply sitting at a computer all day, week after week.

If you have a desk job, you must pay special attention to your spine. The spine is designed for standing, not sitting. Sitting at a desk all day will affect the spine like nothing else. If you work at a desk, set a reminder to go off every 20 or 30 minutes. Whenever the reminder signals you, take at least one minute to stand up, stretch, and walk around your desk. Simple knee bends will work as well as anything. This is vitally important.

Have you ever watched a cat or a dog wake up from a nap? The first thing they do is stretch. Have you ever seen a cat or a dog sit at a computer all day? I didn't think so. We can learn a lot from carefully observing our animal friends.

After just 20 minutes of sitting or lounging, a muscle can shorten by up to one third of its length. For example, the iliopsoas muscle, one of the longest muscles in the body, connects your inner thigh to your bottom five vertebrae. The muscle is designed to keep you standing, and when you sit for an extended period of time, the muscle shrinks. It requires regular stretching to maintain its normal tone and length. If the muscle shortens, it can tug on the vertebrae, causing pain, curvature of the lower back, tilt of the pelvis, and weakness of the hips. Use it or lose it.

If you have a desk job and stand up to stretch every 20 minutes or so, your spine will be in much better shape at the end of the day and in your later years. If you sit at a desk all day without stretching regularly, you will develop degenerative joint disease at some point in your life.

I cannot stress the importance of movement strongly enough. Combined with a healthy diet, regular exercise will prolong your life and fight off disease. It will reduce your risk of heart disease, cancer, and many other illnesses associated with a sedentary lifestyle. I could cite many studies that illustrate the benefits of regular exercise. An example of just one study showing the health benefits of exercise was conducted in Norway which found that lean women who exercise for at least four hours a week have a 72 percent reduction in the risk of breast cancer. On a scale of 1 to 100, 72 is an impressive number! I'd also like to mention the fact that several studies have determined that 30 minutes of daily exercise is as effective as or more effective than prescription antidepressants when it comes to treating depression. Exercise releases endorphins and that makes you feel good.

We all know that regular exercise is healthy. The keyword here is "regular." Set aside 30 minutes every day for your motion therapy, and start out slowly, whether you stretch in bed or walk 10 miles. The important thing is to form the habit. The hard part is getting off the couch and doing it. For that to happen, your mind has to be in the right place. You have to learn how to think right.

10

Think Right

The highly successful MET Right holistic weight loss program is one-third move right, one-third eat right, and one-third think right. All three components are equally important, but if your head's not in the right place, then you won't make the right choices. When you're thinking right you're more likely to choose right.

Do you want to be overweight? I ask my weight loss patients.

"No, of course not," they say.

"Then why do you choose to be overweight?" I ask.

"I don't," they say. "I don't want to be overweight!"

"But you choose to be overweight through the choices you make every day," I explain.

"I can't help myself," they say.

I know.

And I do know. I understand. It's as if they have lost the ability to think for themselves and carry out their will through the choices they make. I feel their pain. In fact, it's not just pain. It's a feeling of hopelessness, I'm out of control, why bother, I can't do anything about it anyway. I was stuck in the same situation for years. I was emotionally as well as physically addicted to junk food.

If you want to lose weight and be healthy, you have to learn how to think right. I wanted to think right. I went through courses and programs to teach myself how to think right. I would do better for a while only to let those negative self thoughts creep back in. But, persistence and determination to change the thoughts you chose to think, does change your thinking. You will succeed. Like anything else, you have to keep practicing this new habit. You have to learn how to think right when you're shopping in the grocery store, ordering at a restaurant, or opening your refrigerator at home. You have to learn how to think right all the time.

Changing your lifestyle and the way you think will not be easy. As a matter of fact, it's one of the hardest things you could possibly do. But it is possible. I see it happening slowly but surely every day.

"Whatever the mind of man can conceive and believe, it can achieve.," said Napoleon Hill, author of *Think and Grow Rich and The Law of Success.* "Thoughts are things! And powerful things at that, when mixed with definiteness of purpose and burning desire, can be translated into riches."

Your weight, your health, your wealth, and your life are determined by your thoughts. To a large extend, your thoughts create your reality.

Here's a thought that might be somewhat confusing or disconcerting at first: Not all of your thoughts are your thoughts. Think about this for a moment.

Well, if they're not my thoughts, then where did they come from? you may be wondering.

Thoughts may be generated by addictive chemicals, microbes in your gut that are craving processed sugar, television commercials, or something your mother said to you when you were three years old.

A cleanse will help you eliminate the physical basis of food addiction. Once you flush out the addictive toxins and unfriendly microorganisms in your gut, you will enjoy a newfound peace of mind. But to counteract other types of "external" or automatic thoughts, you have to change the way you think.

"We are what we are because of the vibrations of thought which we pick up and register through the stimuli of our daily environment," said Hill.

Your thoughts determine your future. Whenever you register a thought, whether consciously or unconsciously, your mind puts energy toward that thought in an effort to make it a reality. That's what the mind does: it turns thoughts into reality. Many people seem to have forgotten this. Many people seem to have forgotten that we humans have great capacity to change.

You *must* take responsibility for your thoughts. Otherwise, you have no control over your future. Until you accept that responsibility, your mind will create a future based on any random thoughts that surface. When you accept responsibility for your thoughts, then you have the power to change your thoughts and your future.

Once you realize this and demand control of your thoughts, your life will change. You will be liberated from your own mind. You will no longer say, "I can't help myself." You *will* help yourself!

The first step in changing the way you think is to carefully monitor your thoughts. You may find this difficult at first. Keep trying. It will become second nature. Pay close attention to your thoughts before you take any type of action. Ask yourself, "Why am I doing this?"

You don't have to act on a thought or impulse just because it surfaces in your mind. Learn to "talk back" to your thoughts.
You can *literally change your mind.*

Sometimes you may find yourself automatically walking toward the kitchen during the commercial break of a television program. You automatically open the cupboard and grab a bag of chips without even thinking about it.

Or you may go grocery shopping with every intention of avoiding junk food only to purchase more chips. How does this happen?

Remember that the midbrain controls your addictions and your emotions. Thus, the midbrain is behind many impulses and automatic behaviors. In our consumer society, we're constantly bombarded by advertisements that attempt to put our midbrain in the driver's seat. When you go grocery shopping, the food manufacturers want your midbrain to make the decisions. You must use your cerebral cortex, the center of higher thinking, to consider the consequences of your actions and override your midbrain when necessary. Your midbrain desires immediate satisfaction in the present moment, but your cerebral cortex has the ability to see into the future.

Monitor your thoughts and behaviors using the intelligent part of your brain. If you feel an urge to walk into the kitchen, examine that urge before acting on it. Catch yourself before you stand up. Ask yourself why you were about to stand up. If your midbrain wanted a bag of chips, use your frontal lobe to consider the consequences. Chips will only lead to weight gain. Ask yourself if you're even really hungry. If you are hungry, consider a healthy snack like an apple.

How to Talk Back to Your Brain

Remember, whenever you register a thought, your brain puts energy toward that thought in an effort to make it a reality. This can be a double-edged sword. If you have positive thoughts, your brain will create a positive reality; however, if you have negative thoughts, your brain will create a negative reality.

"I've trained myself to say 'cancel' in my head whenever I hear a negative thought," says Dr. Jeff Cartwright, my partner in developing the novolife detoxification and cleanse system. Dr. Cartwright and I recently had a discussion about learning how to think right.

"I learned about the 'cancel' method from Mark Victor Hansen, co-creator of the *Chicken Soup for the Soul* series", continues Dr. Cartwright. "If I have a negative thought or hear a negative thought in my environment, I say 'cancel' in my head."

"Sometimes I actually say 'cancel' out-loud just so I can point out the negative thought to others in my environment. For example, if I'm out walking with friends and one of them says, 'Gee, I hope we don't get struck by lightning,' I'll quickly say 'cancel!' to get that negative thought out of my mind, and I'll explain why I said it."

"Negative thoughts are like weeds. You can control those negative thoughts with positive affirmations and visualizations, but you have to catch them early. If you let them slip by for a while, you turn around one day and your garden is full of weeds."

Dr. Cartwright uses affirmations and visualizations to control negative thoughts and encourage positive thoughts. An affirmation is a present-tense, positive statement.

"At any given moment, you're either empowered and in a state of control, or in a state of chaos and low self-esteem," says Dr. Cartwright. "There's rarely an in-between moment. Whenever you're feeling down, use an affirmation to lift yourself back up."

Here are some examples of positive affirmations: *I am a healthy person. I am free. I am loved. I am grateful for my life.*

Remember, the affirmation has to be a positive statement. Telling yourself "I am not fat" will not have the same effect as "I am slim." If you tell yourself, "I am not fat," then your unconscious mind will focus on "fat." Always choose positive words.

If you want to be skinny, then you have to start thinking like a skinny person. If you wake up every morning and think *I'm fat or I wish I weren't fat,* then you'll continue to be fat.

Take a few minutes in the morning to say some positive affirmations to yourself:

I am thin.

I am losing weight.

I am getting stronger.

I am healthy.

"The easiest way to bake a cake is to find someone who can bake a great cake and learn exactly how they do it," points out Dr. Cartwright. If you want to get skinny, then you need to learn how to think like a skinny person. Find a mentor. Find an exercise partner. Seek out people who inspire and motivate you, and spend time with them. Ask them how they got in shape. Ask them how it feels to be skinny. Imagine being thin and enjoying it. If you keep thinking that way, your mind will make it a reality.

"Whenever I hear patients say, 'That's not me!' after looking in the mirror or at a photo, then I know that they're about to lose a lot of weight," says Dr. Cartwright.

It can be difficult to maintain positive thoughts in our crazy society.

The media bombards us with images of negativity. The best way to avoid those negative images is to turn off your television. Change your environment. Get off the couch. Get out there and *live.* I still watch television sometimes, but I try to avoid any negative, depressing content.

"I don't watch the news," Dr. Cartwright tells me. "If something important happens, I always hear about it from other people. I don't watch negative shows, either, and I only read books and magazines that are going to uplift me and keep my thoughts positive."

Positive thinking will attract positive people into your life and help you to be a happier, healthier person. Positive thinking is a great source of healing and an agent of change. Your thoughts affect your body in a very real way.

The mind-body connection is no longer a secret shared only by Eastern mystics. Western science has accepted the validity of the mind-body connection. One medical study found that optimistic patients recovered more quickly after heart surgery. In fact, pessimistic patients died at twice the rate of optimistic patients!

Your body reacts to your thoughts on a cellular level. Negative thinking can easily disrupt the delicate biochemistry within your cells. If your mind thinks that you are sick, then your body will feel sick. If your mind thinks that you are fat, you will be fat.

Whenever a negative thought surfaces, cancel it! If you think, "I might as well order pizza tonight because I'm already 30 pounds overweight," cancel that thought immediately. Replace it with a positive thought: "I'm going to have salmon and steamed vegies tonight because I'm losing 30 pounds." You have the power to change your way of thinking!

When you're shopping in the grocery store, don't think about all the unhealthy foods that you're *not* going to buy (or you just might end up buying them). Instead, think about all the healthy foods that you will buy. Focus on the positives.

Negative thought: *I'm not going to buy junk food.*

Positive thoughts: I'm going to buy only healthy whole foods created by God, not designed by engineers in a laboratory. I'm going to buy only foods with natural ingredients that I can pronounce.

This is how I'm trying to think, and I find myself buying less and less junk food that I had no intention of buying. When you are in control of your thoughts and actions, grocery shopping is a creative, liberating experience. I try to find fruits and vegetables that I've never eaten before. You don't have to buy the same old junk food. Sometimes we go shopping with the kids and grandkids and it's a fun experience creating a delicious, healthy menu. It's even more fun to go to a local farmer's market and create a fresh meal for the evening.

Visualize Your Future

Self-image is critical. If you see yourself as an overweight individual, then you'll carry yourself as an overweight individual. You'll dress differently. Your posture will slump. You won't be motivated to move right. You will have a negative self-image.

Many of my overweight patients have a self-image that's much worse than reality. If you have a negative self-image, start by looking in the mirror. See the real you. Smile at yourself. Accept yourself. Now begin to visualize your health. Visualize a healthy body, and think about what you must do to maintain that healthy body.

You can even visualize the interior of your body! During your cleanse, visualize the toxins exiting your body. Visualize your white blood cells gobbling up excess debris and germs. Visualize your fat cells melting away and disappearing.

"In most cases, the biggest obstacle to weight loss is a lack of self-esteem," says Dr. Cartwright.

Jack Canfield, the other co-creator of *Chicken Soup for the Soul,* said, "Too many times people are thinking a thought like, 'I want to be my perfect body weight of 185 pounds.' But they look at the scale and they see 205 and they think, 'But I'll never make it,' … so they feel bad."

Instead of giving into negative thinking patterns, cancel them and find the positive aspect of the situation. You have the ability to lose weight, get healthy, and make your life better. You can do something about it. Focus on what you need to do. If you continue to carry around negative thoughts, you'll live into them and they will remain your reality.

The law of attraction, popularized by the film *The Secret,* states that "like attracts like." If you have positive thoughts and feelings, you'll attract positive thoughts and feelings into your life. If you have negative thoughts and feelings, you'll attract negativity into your life.

There's nothing magical about the law of attraction. It's completely logical. Our future is determined by our choices and actions, which are determined by our thoughts and feelings. When you're thinking about your future, you're actually creating your future. As Robert Anton Wilson wrote in *Prometheus Rising*, "The future exists first in imagination, then in will, then in reality."

You have to visualize your future and act to make it happen. Otherwise, you're living your life at the whim of a whimsical universe.

Set Goals and Reward Yourself

After you visualize your future, set goals to make it happen. Write down your goals. If you want to lose 30 pounds in six months, write it down. Get out your calendar and mark the date. Figure out how many pounds you need to lose each week. Let's see . . . You'd need to lose 1.25 pounds a week. Write it down. Whenever you feel discouraged, look at your goals. Focus on your goals.

You have to track your progress. Otherwise, you might completely forget about the goals! Weigh yourself at least once a week. When you meet your goals, reward yourself. Celebrate! You deserve it!

When you find yourself slipping - if you gain a couple of pounds after a weekend of cheating - hold yourself accountable, but don't beat yourself up over it. That's negativity speaking!

Nobody's perfect. The 12 steps of Alcoholics Anonymous are followed by an important qualifying statement: "No one among us has been able to maintain anything like perfect adherence to these principles. We are not saints. The point is that we were willing to grow along spiritual lines. The principles we have set down are guides to progress. We claim spiritual progress rather than spiritual perfection."

You don't have to be perfect. Your body weight will naturally fluctuate. You will gain a few pounds here and there. Don't get discouraged. You know how to lose those pounds: do a mini-cleanse to reset your system. Don't allow negative thoughts to creep back into your mind.

Again, I know that it can be hard to remain positive in a society that can be so overtly negative at times. Whenever you're feeling stressed or depressed, get up and get moving. Go for a walk. Exercise releases endorphins in your brain that will make you feel better; remember it can be more effective than antidepressant medication.

If you think that you may be clinically depressed, talk to a counselor. A counselor will help you let go of guilt and resentment. You can't live your life in the past, but you can't ignore the past, either. Learn from the past without clinging to it. Forgive yourself for past mistakes and focus on avoiding the same mistakes in the future. Forgive others as well. Resentment breeds negativity. Everybody makes mistakes. Nobody is perfect.

Laugh frequently. He who laughs, lasts. Laughing burns calories and lifts the spirit. Watch the comedy channel instead of the news.

Spend time with children and animals. You can learn a lot from them. Plus, studies show that owning a pet can reduce stress, lower blood pressure, and boost immunity. Unfortunately, I can't say that having kids reduces stress, but it is a very rewarding experience in its own right. And, there's no better way to get the best stress reducer in life, grandkids!

Many people find that volunteer work helps them to maintain positive thoughts. Service work will help you put your own problems in perspective, and it feels good to help others.

Finally, several studies show that prayer and meditation boost immunity as well as emotional well-being. If you're thinking, "I don't have time for prayer or meditation," then you're one of the people who definitely needs to make time! You don't need much time. You can say your prayers at night before you fall asleep. Focus on gratitude. Think about all the wonderful things in your life. Even if you are not a religious person, take a few minutes each day to think about those things in your life for which you are grateful. I've had patients tell me they don't have anything to be thankful for in their life. I remind them they can be thankful for the bed they are laying in, for the air-conditioning they are enjoying, or for weather outside (no matter what the weather is). When you start listing you will find the things to be thankful for far outweigh the negatives in your life.

I also do a few deep breathing exercises every night. When you focus on your breath, you're telling your brain to relax. Deep breathing will lower your stress and blood pressure and help you lose weight. Cortisol is a hormone released due to stress. Elevated levels of cortisol can lead to weight gain.

You don't have to sit in the lotus position and chant "om" for half an hour to benefit from deep breathing exercises. You can do simple deep breathing exercises anytime, anywhere – whenever you need to relax and release some stress.

My favorite deep breathing exercise is the 4-7-8 breathing technique. I learned this from Dr. Andrew Weil in one of his DVD programs, and I've been using it ever since then. You will feel the benefits immediately. It's simple, easy to learn, and you can do it anywhere (even at work). Sit up straight and slowly inhale through your nostrils for 4 seconds. Hold the breath for 7 seconds. Imagine the oxygen rejuvenating your cells. Exhale slowly through your mouth for 8 seconds. Try to completely empty your lungs by the count of 8. Repeat this several times until you feel relaxed. It won't take long.

Deep breathing exercises will not only help you relax, but they will also stimulate your cardiovascular and lymphatic systems, helping your body to release toxins and fat. Other relaxation techniques include meditation, yoga, tai chi, and qi gong. Consider taking a class. Try something new. You have a long life ahead of you, and you don't want to keep doing the same things over and over again!

People come to see me because they want to lose weight or eliminate pain, and it gives me the opportunity to teach them how to live longer, healthier lives. That's my mission. If you cleanse your body of toxins and start eating a diet rich in whole, unrefined fruits and vegetables, there's no reason that you can't live a long, healthy, happy life of 100 years or more.

I know what it feels like to be fat. I was the "Fat Boy." Now, I'm slim and healthy, and I'm looking forward to the long life ahead of me.

Change is difficult, but it doesn't have to be painful. If you like going out to eat with your friends, then go out to eat with your friends. *When you get hungry, eat!* But eat healthy foods that will promote health and well-being rather than pain, inflammation, weight gain, and disease. Eat whole foods with high nutrient densities - the foods that God intended for us to eat.

Get moving. Just move. Thirty minutes of movement above and beyond your normal daily routine. (Make it a habit, remember forty days.)

You are the creator of your future, and you always have a choice.

If you're ready to lose weight now, go look at yourself in the mirror. Accept yourself. Visualize what you want and how you're going to get it. Write down your goals. You may even want to take a "before" photo of yourself. Save it as a souvenir. You'll be proud of your journey.

Move Right, Eat Right, *Think* Right.
            It's time for a new beginning!

References

Chapter 1
http://www.nci.nih.gov/newscenter/benchmarks-vol4-issue3/page1

Chapter 2
http://oem.bmj.com/cgi/reprint/64/9/626.pdf

http://bastyrcenter.org/content/view/313/&page=

http://www.medicalnewstoday.com/articles/125782.php

http://ohioline.osu.edu/hyg-fact/2000/2157.html

Aiello AE, Marshall B, Levy SB, Della-Latta P, Larson E (2004). "Relationship between triclosan and susceptibilities of bacteria isolated from hands in the community". Antimicrob. Agents Chemother. 48 (8): 2973–9

Aiello AE, Marshall B, Levy SB, Della-Latta P, Larson E (2004). "Relationship between triclosan and susceptibilities of bacteria isolated from hands in the community". Antimicrob. Agents Chemother. 48 (8): 2973–9.

Dons Bach KW, Walker M. Drinking Water. Huntingdon Beach, CA: Int'l

Institute of Natural Health Sciences, 1981.

http://www.foodnews.org/EWG-shoppers-guide-download-final.pdf

http://www.ajcn.org/cgi/content/full/79/4/537

Department of Health and Human Services, Report on All Adverse Reactions in the Adverse Reaction Monitoring System, (February 25 and 28, 1994).

http://www.wnho.net/the_ecologist_aspartame_report.html

New Scientist -18 September 1986, Ian Anderson

Ainsleigh, H. Gordon. Beneficial effects of sun exposure on cancer mortality. Preventive Medicine, Vol. 22, February 1993, pp. 132-40

http://www.naturalnews.com/024993_mercury_the_FDA_mercury_fillings.html

Occupational and environmental health by Barry S. Levy, David H. Wegman, Sherry L. Baron, Rosemary K. Sokas. p 22

http://www.epa.gov/iedweb00/pubs/insidest.html

The Complete Organic Pregnancy by Deirdre Dolan, Alexandra Zissu

http://www.ewg.org/reports/rocketwater

http://environmentallegal.blogs.com/sholzer/2008/11/federal-epa-will-not-regulate-perchlorate.html

http://www.environmentalhealthnews.org/newscience/2007/2007-1109calafatetal.html

http://www.abcnews.go.com/Health/Story?id=5809117&page=1

http://www.cosmeticsdatabase.com/

http://www.forbes.com/2008/12/16/toys-product-safety-biz-commerce-cx_wp_1216toxictoys.html

http://www.usatoday.com/news/health/2008-09-14-drugs-flush-water_N.html

http://www.medicine.org/profiles/blogs/acetaminophen-overdoses

http://www.cancer.org/docroot/PED/content/PED_1_3x_Known_and_Probable_Carcinogens.asp

Tareke E, Rydberg P. et al. (2002). "Analysis of acrylamide, a carcinogen formed in heated foodstuffs". J. Agric. Food. Chem. 50 (17): 4998–5006

http://www.thelancet.com/journals/lancet/article/PIIS0140673607613063/abstract

Rowe KS, Rowe KJ. Synthetic food coloring and behavior: a dose response effect in a double-blind, placebo-controlled, repeated-measures study. J Pediatr. 1994 Nov;125(5 Pt 1):691-8.

O'Brien, Robyn. The Unhealthy Truth: How Our Food Is Making Us Sick and What We Can Do About It.

http://www.huffingtonpost.com/christine-escobar/the-tale-of-rbgh-milk-mon_b_170823.html

http://www.preventcancer.com/press/releases/july8_98.htm

http://www.naturalnews.com/021784.html

http://www.cornallergens.com/list/corn-allergen-list.php

http://www.scientificamerican.com/article.cfm?id=that-burger-youre-eating-is-mostly-corn

http://www.foodrevolution.org/grassfedbeef.htm

Daniel Sheehan and Daniel Doerge, "Goitrogenic and Estrogenic Activity of Soy Isoflavones," Environmental Health Perspectives 110, suppl. 3 (June 2002): 349-53.

http://jn.nutrition.org/cgi/reprint/119/2/211.pdf

Netherwood et al.., "Assessing the Survival of Transgenic Plant DNA in the Human Gastrointestinal Tract," Nature Biotechnology 22 (2004).

http://www.seedsofdeception.com/Public/BuyingNon-GMO/index.cfm

http://www.drlam.com/opinion/toxic_food.asp

http://www.medicalnewstoday.com/articles/68822.php

Chapter 3

Shore SA, Fredberg JJ. Obesity, smooth muscle, and airway hyperresponsiveness. J Allergy Clin Immunol. 2005;115:925-927.

http://www.wrongdiagnosis.com/a/asthma/deaths.htm

http://www.medscape.com/viewarticle/583629

Eberhart MS, Ogden C, Engelgau M, Cadwell B, Hedley AA, Saydah SH (November 2004). "Prevalence of overweight and obesity among adults with diagnosed diabetes—United States, 1988-1994 and 1999-2002". MMWR Morb. Mortal. Wkly. Rep. 53 (45): 1066–8

http://www.usc.edu/hsc/info/pr/hmm/04winter/fat.html

Arlan Rosenbloom, Janet H Silverstein (2003). Type 2 Diabetes in Children and Adolescents: A Clinician's Guide to Diagnosis, Epidemiology, Pathogenesis, Prevention, and Treatment. American Diabetes Association,U.S.. pp. 1

Lang IA, Galloway TS, Scarlett A, et al. (September 2008). "Association of urinary bisphenol A concentration with medical disorders and laboratory abnormalities in adults". JAMA 300 (11): 1303–10.

http://www.diabetes.org/diabetes-statistics/dangerous-toll.jsp

http://www.the-natural-path.com/food-that-lowers-cholesterol.html

Ford ES, Giles WH, Dietz WH (2002). Prevalence of metabolic syndrome among US adults: findings from the third National Health and Nutrition Examination Survey. JAMA 287(3):356-359

http://www.webmd.com/back-pain/news/20090209/obesity-a-pain-in-the-back

Food Addiction by Kay Sheppard. Health Communications. 1993.

http://www.prevention.com/cda/article/bye-bye%20-blues/346d72e50d803110VgnVCM10000013281eac____/nutrition.recipes/nutrition.basics/foods.for.specific.conditions/mood.boosters/

http://www.ehjournal.net/content/8/1/2

http://www.psychologytoday.com/articles/200304/vitamin-b-key-energy

Gordon C, Feldman H, Sinclair L et al. Prevalence of Vitamin D deficiency among healthy infants and toddlers: Archives Pediatrics and Adolescent Medicine 2008:162(6):505-512

http://www.sciencedaily.com/releases/2008/02/080217211802.htm

http://ucsdnews.ucsd.edu/newsrel/science/cancer07.asp

Friedenreich CM. Physical activity and cancer prevention: From observational to intervention research. Cancer Epidemiology, Biomarkers and Prevention 2001; 10(4):287–301.

Parker ED, Folsom AR. *Intentional weight loss and incidence of obesity-related cancers: The Iowa Women's Health Study. International Journal of Obesity and Related Metabolic Disorders* 2003; 27(12):1447–1452.

Whitlock G, Lewington S, Sherliker P, et al. (March 2009). "Body-mass index and cause-specific mortality in 900 000 adults: collaborative analyses of 57 prospective studies". *Lancet* 373 (9669): 1083–96.

http://emedicine.medscape.com/article/123702-overview

http://www.cdc.gov/obesity/data/index.html

http://jn.nutrition.org/cgi/content/abstract/139/3/623

Chapter 4

http://www.myaddiction.com/education/articles/sex_statistics.html

http://www.usatoday.com/news/health/2007-07-09-food-addiction_N.htm

http://jn.nutrition.org/cgi/content/full/133/3/835S

http://healthfieldmedicare.suite101.com/article.cfm/the_brainfood_connection

http://www.cinchouse.com/MindBody/HealthBeauty/tabid/77/articleType/ ArticleView/articleId/85/Americas-Food-Addiction.aspx

http://www.npr.org/templates/story/story.php?storyId=94761977

Gabriel Cousens. *There is a Cure for Diabetes.*

Adreas Moritz. *Timeless Secrets of Health & Rejuvenation.*

http://ajpregu.physiology.org/cgi/content/abstract/00195.2008v1

J. Blundell et al., *The Lancet, Paradoxical effects of an intense sweetener (aspartame) on appetite,* vol.1, 1986, pp.1092-1093.

http://www.naturodoc.com/library/nutrition/aspartame.htm

http://www.ncbi.nlm.nih.gov/pubmed/18800291?dopt=Abstract

http://www.cspinet.org/nah/4_00/stevia.html

http://www.greenermagazine.com/articlesMSG.html

http://insulinresistanceca.com/msg-increases-insulin-in-your-blood/

http://www.laynetworks.com/TYPES-OF-MOTIVATION.html

http://weightloss.about.com/b/2007/08/25/have-your-say-3.htm

Chapter 5

Digestive Wellness: Completely Revised and Updated Third Edition by Elizabeth Lipski

Yongchaiyudha S, Rungpitarangsi V, Bunyapraphatsara N, Chokechaijaroenporn O. (1996) *Antidiabetic activity of Aloe vera L juice. I. Clinical trial in new* cases of diabetes mellitus. *Phytomedicine 3: 241–243; Bunyapraphatsara N, Yongchaiyudha S, Rungpitarangsi V, Chokechaijaroenporn O. (1996) Antidiabetic activity of Aloe vera L juice. II. Clinical trial in diabetes mellitus patients in combination with glibenclamide. Phytomedicine 3: 245–248. Nassiff HA, Fajardo F, Velez F. (1993) Effecto del aloe sobre la hiperlipidemia en pacientes refractarios a la dieta (The effect of Aloe in the diet in hyperlipidemic patients) Rev Cuba Med Gen Integr 9:43–51.*

Savendahl L, Mar MH, Underwood LE, Zeisel SH. Prolonged fasting in humans results in diminished plasma choline concentrations but does not cause liver dysfunction. Am J Clin Nutr. 1997;66(3):622-5.

Anderson RA. Chromium in the prevention and control of diabetes. Diabetes and Metabolism . 2000;26(1)22-27.

Gordon JB. An easy and inexpensive way to lower cholesterol? West J Med . 1991 Mar;154(3):352.

Anderson RA. Effects of chromium on body composition and weight loss . Nutr Rev . 1998;56(9):266-270.

Levine J, Barak Y, Kofman O, and Belmaker RH. Follow-up and relapse analysis of an inositol study of depression. Isr J Psychiatry Relat Sci 32(1): 14–21, 1995.

http://www.drcolbert.com/cont_articles.php?action=full&artcat=3&aid=67

http://www.detoxification.ws/disease-healing/fasting-for-blood-parasites-and-candida

http://www.drcolbert.com/cont_articles.php?action=full&artcat=3&aid=67

http://www.yogamag.net/archives/1981/emay81/jap.shtml

Chapter 6

Berenson, GS, SR Srinivasan, TA Nicklas. 1998. Association between multiple cardiovascular risk factors and atherosclerosis in children and young adults. N. Eng. J. Med. 338: 1650-56.

Joel Fuhrman, MD. Eat to Live: The Revolutionary Formula for Fast and Sustained Weight Loss. 2003. Little, Brown and Company. P 38.

http://www.whfoods.org/genpage.php?tname=foodspice&dbid=38#healthbenefits

http://www.whfoods.com/genpage.php?tname=foodspice&dbid=43

http://www.essortment.com/all/whatbokchoych_rgsv.htm

http://www.fitsugar.com/node/167874/results

http://www.theworldwidegourmet.com/products/vegetables/boston-lettuce-or-butter-lettuce/

http://www.whfoods.com/genpage.php?tname=foodspice&dbid=9

http://www.whfoods.com/genpage.php?tname=foodspice&dbid=19

Michael Murray ND and Joseph Pizzorno ND. Encyclopedia of Natural Medicine, Revised Second Edition.

Agriculture Fact Book 2001-2002. U.S. Department of Agriculture. March 2003. 15 (pdf).

Rob Stein. "Daily Red Meat Raises Chances Of Dying Early." Washington Post. 24 March 2009.

http://www.cspinet.org/new/cheese.html

http://www.deflame.com/Diet/tabid/83/Default.aspx

Colgan, Michael. The New Nutrition.

http://www.welikeitraw.com/rawfood/2009/06/dr-robert-young-you-are-what-you-eat-and-what-you-think.html

Joel Fuhrman. Eat to Live. P 124.

Innis, SA. 1991. Essential fatty acids in growth and development. Prog. Lipd Res. 30: 39-103.

Siguel, EN and RH Lerman. 1994. Altered fatty acid metabolism in patients with angiographic ally documented coronary artery disease. Metabolism 43: 982-83; Adams, PB, S Lawson, A Sanigorski and AJ Sinclair. 1996. Arachidonic acid to eicosapentaenoic acid ration in blood correlates positively with clinical symptoms of depression. Lipids 31 Supp: s157-61; Rose, DP. 1997. Effects of dietary fatty acids on breast and prostate cancers: evidence from in vitro experiments and animal studies. Am. J. Clin. Nutr. 66: 1513s-22s.

http://www.cnn.com/2009/HEALTH/expert.q.a/04/10/water.losing.weight.jampolis/index.html

http://news.bbc.co.uk/2/hi/uk_news/england/tyne/7067226.stm

http://www.timesonline.co.uk/tol/news/uk/health/article2753446.ece

http://www.bfa.com.au/_files/20070327_Organic%20IS%20Healthier.pdf

http://www.webmd.com/food-recipes/news/20060110/organic-food-worth-money

http://www.beyondhealth.com/milk.aspx

http://www.milksucks.com/osteo.asp

http://www.thepaleodiet.com/faqs/

Chapter 7

http://www.leslietaylor.net/herbal/herbal.htm

Heitzman, M.E., Neto, C.C., Winiarz, E., Vaisberg, A.J. & Hammon, G.B. (2005). Ethnobotany, phytochemistry and pharmacology of Uncaria (Rubiaceae).

Phytochemistry, 66(1), 5-29

http://www.time.com/time/magazine/article/0,9171,1191810,00.html

Huffman MA (May 2003). "Animal self-medication and ethno-medicine: exploration and exploitation of the medicinal properties of plants". Proc Nutr Soc 62 (2): 371–81.

Hutchings MR, Athanasiadou S, Kyriazakis I, Gordon IJ (May 2003). "Can animals use foraging behavior to combat parasites?". Proc Nutr Soc. 62 (2): 361

http://www.biomesonline.com/monographs/medicine.html

http://newsroom.ucla.edu/portal/ucla/fruits-vegetables-and-teas-may-51210.aspx

http://library.thinkquest.org/24206/quotes.html

http://www.litalee.com/shopcontent.asp?type=HowEnzymesHeal

Gillman et al. Journal of the American Medical Association. 1995;273;1113

Gaziano et al. Annals of Epidemiology 1995;5:255 and Colditz et al. American Journal of Clinical Nutrition 1985;41:32

Giovannucci et al. Journal of the National Cancer Institute 1995;87:1767

Cohen, JH, AR Kristal, JL Stanford. 200. Fruit and vegetable intakes and prostate cancer risk. J. Nat. Cancer Inst. 92 (1): 61-68.

Seddon et al. Journal of the American Medical Association. 1994;272:1413

Fuhrman, Joel. Eat to Live. P 49

Nelson, NJ. 1996. Is chemoprevention research overrated or underrated? Primary Care and Cancer 16 98): 29.

Fuhrman, Joel. Eat to Live. p 58.

http://whfoods.org/genpage.php?tname=foodspice&dbid=38#nutritionalprofile

Zhao H, Lin J, Grossman HB, Hernandez LM, Dinney CP and Wu X. Dietary isothiocyanates, GSTM1, GSTT1, NAT2 polymorphisms and bladder cancer risk. International Journal of Cancer. 120: 2208-2213, 2007

Voorrips LE, Goldbohm RA, et al. Vegetable and fruit consumption and risks of colon and rectal cancer in a prospective cohort study: The Netherlands Cohort Study on Diet and Cancer. Am J Epidemiol. 2000 Dec 1;152(11):1081-92. 2000. PMID:11117618.

Zhao B, Seow A, et al. Dietary isothiocyanates, glutathione S-transferase

-M1, -T1 polymorphisms and lung cancer risk among Chinese women in Singapore. Cancer Epidemiol Biomarkers Prev. 2001 Oct;10(10):1063-7. 2001. PMID:11588132.

http://www.igonutrition.com/2008_03_23_archive.html

Maiyoh GK, Kuh JE, Casaschi A, Theriault AG. Cruciferous indole-3-carbinol inhibits apolipoprotein B secretion in HepG2 cells. J Nutr. 2007 Oct;137(10):2185-9. 2007. PMID:17884995.

http://whfoods.org/genpage.php?tname=foodspice&dbid=61#healthbenefits

http://www.medicinenet.com/script/main/art.asp?articlekey=564

Lu QY, Hung JC, Heber D, et al. Inverse associations between plasma lycopene and other carotenoids and prostate cancer. Cancer Epidemiol Biomarkers Prev. 2001 Jul;10(7):749-56 2001.

Yuan JM, Stram DO, Arakawa K, Lee HP, Yu MC. Dietary cryptoxanthin and reduced risk of lung cancer: the Singapore Chinese Health Study. Cancer Epidemiol Biomarkers Prev. 2003 Sep;12(9):890-8. 2003.

Ishida BK, Chapman MH. A comparison of carotenoid content and total antioxidant activity in catsup from several commercial sources in the United States. J Agric Food Chem. 2004 Dec 29;52(26):8017-20. 2004. PMID:15612790.

Canene-Adams K, Lindshield BL, Wang S, Jeffery EH, Clinton SK, Erdman JW Jr. Combinations of tomato and broccoli enhance antitumor activity in dunning r3327-h prostate adenocarcinomas. Cancer Res. 2007 Jan 15;67(2):836-43. Epub 2007 Jan 9. 2007. PMID:17213256.

http://whfoods.org/genpage.php?tname=foodspice&dbid=8

Andres-Lacueva C, Shukitt-Hale B, Galli RL, Jauregui O, Lamuela-Raventos RM, Joseph JA. Anthocyanins in aged blueberry-fed rats are found centrally and may enhance memory. Nutr Neurosci. 2005 Apr;8(2):111-20. 2005. PMID:16053243.

Yi W, Fischer J, Krewer G, Akoh CC. Phenolic compounds from blueberries can inhibit colon cancer cell proliferation and induce apoptosis. J Agric Food Chem. 2005 Sep 7;53(18):7320-9. 2005. PMID:16131149.

Wu X, Beecher GR, Holden JM, Haytowitz DB, Gebhardt SE, Prior RL. Concentrations of Anthocyanins in Common Foods in the United States and Estimation of Normal Consumption. J Agric Food Chem. 2006 May 31;54(11):4069-4075. 2006. PMID:16719536.

Chapter 8
Fuhrman, Joel. Eat to Live. P 83.

Chen, JT, TC Campbell, J Li, R Peto. 1990. Diet, lifestyle and mortality in China: a study of the caracteristics of 65 Chinese counties. Oxford: Oxford University Press; Ithaca, NY: Cornell University Press; Beijing;: Peoples Medical Publishing House, p. 894.

Kasiske, BL, JD Lakatua, JZ Ma, TA Louis. 1998. A meta-anaylsis of the effects of dietary protein restriction on the rate of decline in renal function. Am. J. Kidney Dis. 31 (6): 954-61.

Pedrini, MT, AS Levey, J Lau, TC Chalmers, PH Wang. 1996. The effect of dietary protein on the progression of diabetic and no diabetic renal disease: a meta-analysis. Ann. Intern. Med. 124 (7) 627-32.

Fuhrman, Joel, eat to Live p 93.

La Vecchia, C, A Tavani. 1998. Fruit and vegetables, and human cancer. Eur. J. Cancer Prev. 7 (1): 3-8.

Key, TJA, M Thorogood, PN Appleby, and ML Burr. 1996. Dietary habits and mortality in 11000 vegetarians and health conscious people: results of a 17-year followup. BMJ 313: 775-79.

Karra, Cindy: Shape Up America! Reveals The Truth About Dieters, Shape Up America! (by former U.S. Surgeon General C. Everett Koop)

Fuhrman, Joel. Eat to Live. P 41.

Fuhrman, Joel. Eat to Live. P 101.

http://www.webmd.com/diet/news/20070411/diets-dont-work-long-term

http://sportsmedicine.about.com/od/sportsnutrition/a/060304.htm

Chapter 9

Galileo and the Birth of Modern Science, by Stephen Hawking, American Heritage's Invention & Technology, Spring 2009, Vol. 24, No. 1, p. 36.

Talanian, JL, SDR Galloway, GJF Heigenhauser, A Bonen, LL Spriet. Two weeks of high intensity aerobic interval training increase the capacity for fat oxidation during exercise in women. J Appl Physiol 102: 1439-1447, 2007

Burgomaster, KA, SC Hughes, GJF Heigenhauser, SN Bradwell, MJ Gibala. Six sessions of sprint interval training increases muscle oxidative potential and cycle endurance capacity in humans. J Appl Physiol 98: 1985-1990, 2005.

http://www.selfgrowth.com/articles/Chiropractic_And_Spinal_Health.html

Chapter 10

Thune, I, T Brenn, E Lund, M Gaard. Physical Activity and the Risk of Breast Cancer. The New England Journal of Medicine. 336: 1269-1275.

http://en.wikiquote.org/wiki/Napoleon_Hill

http://www.medicinenet.com/script/main/art.asp?articlekey=87828

http://www.webmd.com/hypertension-high-blood-pressure/features/health-benefits-of-pets

http://nccam.nih.gov/news/newsletter/2005_winter/prayer.htm

http://stress.about.com/od/stresshealth/a/weightgain.htm

LaVergne, TN USA
19 February 2010
173730LV00001B/24/P